God's Plan for Wellness

God's Plan for Wellness

Kathleen LeSage

CrossLink Publishing

CrossLink Publishing
558 E. Castle Pines Pkwy, Ste B4117
Castle Rock, CO 80108
www.crosslinkpublishing.com

Ordering Information:
Quantity sales. Special discounts are available on quantity purchases by corporations, associations, and others. For details, contact the "Special Sales Department" at the address above.

God's Plan for Wellness/LeSage —1st ed.
ISBN 978-1-63357-118-1
Library of Congress Control Number: 2017949915

Front cover photo: James T. Le Sage, Jr.

For James & LeAnne.

The two biggest blessings of my life.

I love you both with all that is in me and I always will!

Wellness is the health of mind, body and spirit. All three have to be in line together to really define a total being of wellness. One can be at a healthy weight and exercise regularly, but if that same person is in a stressful life situation or not feeding the spirit, the other areas need to be focused on and brought into alignment in order to experience complete wellness.
—Kathleen LeSage

From the "Destination Spa Group: Summer Words of Wellness" on Spafinder

Contents

Acknowledgements

The biggest acknowledgement goes to Jimmy LeSage, my husband, father of my children, business partner, and gift from God. It truly was Divine Intervention that brought our paths together in Naples, and the blessings that have followed over the past fifteen years have been amazing. Thank you for believing in me, supporting me, helping me follow my dreams, teaching me about wellness, letting me be the mother I always dreamed I could be, and most importantly, loving me and marrying me at a period in my life when I was not at my best. You truly were a godsend, and I cherish the life we have together.

A huge dose of gratitude goes to my parents, who are now both in heaven. I will forever be grateful for being raised in a Christian home and for the sacrifices they made to give me a Christian education while growing up in the suburbs of Washington, DC.

I would also like to thank Dr. Sears and the entire team at the Dr. Sears Wellness Institute. You were my go-to author/pediatrician when my children were babies and I needed sound advice. It has been a pleasure being a Certified Health Coach through your organization, and I continue to learn from the Institute the latest research in wellness and health.

Thank you to my dad's twin sister (and my favorite aunt), Audrey Nesmith, who has always been a source of encouragement from the time I was a teenager. Thank you for listening to me go on and on about my children with the interest and patience that only a grandparent could ever have.

Pastor Lon Solomon, thank you for meeting with me on March 26, 2002. Your wise counseling set me on a path that put me where I am today.

Lastly, thank you to Roger Miller. From the first huge hug you gave me in your office in northern Virginia, I knew you would be more than just an advisor. Throughout my entire adult life you have been more like a father to me. Thank you for your wisdom over the past several decades and the encouragement to move to Naples. My life would not have taken the turn it did and my family would not be where it is today without your advice. Your impact on my life has been even bigger than your hugs!

God bless you all!

Introduction

My own journey into health and wellness has been an unlikely one. However, looking back, I can see the hand of God in every step of the way. Even when I wasn't looking toward God, He was there.

I grew up a chunky child. Healthy food was not plentiful in my home. With the exception of a bag of apples that my mom would wash and put in a bowl in the center of the kitchen table, most of our vegetables and fruits were canned and loaded with sugar or salt. I had one grandfather who worked for Wonder Bread and another grandfather who worked for Nabisco. My parents were raised on a mountain of processed food, and I was too. I could have been the poster child of a white flour diet. My lunches were often two pieces of white Wonder Bread with some sort of processed meat in the middle, chips, a Twinkie or a package of Little Debbies, and one of the apples from the bowl on the table (which often tasted terrible and got thrown in the trash after the first bite).

I do also have to mention that my grandfather who worked as a baker at Wonder Bread in Washington, DC also had a huge vegetable garden that he would tend to during the weekends in the summer. His garden was at my grandparents' little cottage on the water in southern Maryland. We would spend summers there and feast on the produce my grandfather would grow, along with the fish and crabs we would catch off his dock on the water. My family was often running around outside, swimming, and riding bikes. Looking back, I can now make the connection between that lifestyle and how much healthier I felt during the summer.

But I was still pretty heavy, even with the healthier fare and increased exercise. Sweets were never far off; there was always a box of something packaged from Hostess, Little Debbie, or Nabisco within arm's reach. I was never known to eat "just one."

It wasn't until my teenage years that I tried to take control of my weight. And it wasn't because I was concerned about my health. It was only because I wanted to lose weight to try out for things that one would need to be fit and trim for. I did spend a few years modeling in Washington, DC, for downtown department stores, and I was fortunate to hold a few pageant titles (Miss Georgetown - DC, Miss Maryland Teen, and a few others), but I got slim and trim through starvation diets, body wraps, or whatever other fad was all the rage to lose weight and lose weight quick.

It was during these "pageant years" that I developed extremely unhealthy habits. I am not saying everyone did what I did in this industry. There were many young women who were fit and trim because they also competed in sports or in dance. I was not naturally fit. I did crazy things to fit into a certain size, with no regard for my health. My health was not even on my radar.

During this time in the early '90s, I had the fortunate opportunity to meet Cheryl Prewitt Salem, a former Miss America who had a Christian ministry and was also a talented vocalist. She had written books about her life (which included a miraculous healing) and traveled to share her testimony. She was the one who planted the seeds of exercise and healthy eating in me, although those seeds would take many years to sprout.

At this time, I did a Bible study on the book of Esther and became fascinated with how long beauty treatments had been around. I became very interested in the beauty industry and considered having a career in it. However, keep in mind, this was about beauty, NOT wellness. My interest was not in doing what was healthy for my body; it was just simply to look good, feed my vanity, and enjoy a few spa treatments. It didn't last long. Having been born and raised in the Washington, DC area, where good jobs in the government and private sector are plentiful, I was encouraged by my family to "get a real job."

Have you ever heard the saying, "Life is what happens when you are busy making other plans"? Well, that's what happened to me. I ended up realizing that my best bet at having a career and continuing my education would be to get a job at a company in DC. While working during the day in an office, commuting in DC traffic a few hours a day, and attending school at night at the University of Maryland, the pounds crept on as I settled into a sedentary lifestyle. By the time I hit thirty years old, I weighed 240 pounds.

I only share these details to give you a little glimpse of how I went from actually competing in (and winning a few) pageants and participating in modeling assignments to having to buy my clothes at a plus-sized store and squeezing into an airplane seat. I'm not someone who has always been into sports and health. I'm a real woman with real struggles. But I believe that these experiences (and I am glossing over the entire story of the weight gain; that is a separate book on its own) gave me the understanding and the empathy to help people who feel like they are so far down an unhealthy path that they might not ever get healthy again.

Completing my training as a certified health coach and running one of the top wellness retreats in the country isn't an automatic ticket to being healthy. It is a lifestyle choice I deal with and struggle with every day. My husband started the business forty years ago, and we have been running it together for the last fifteen years. To this day, most of my responsibilities running the business have to do with marketing and administration. It is a daily fight to find the time to go on a hike, stretch, and make wise eating choices.

This book contains real tips and tricks I have found to help real people. Over the past fifteen years, I have been entrenched in wellness and health. I have also seen how far out in left field some of the ideas can be. God has a plan for all of us. God has a plan for the health and wellness of His people. He outlined it in His Word. It is never too late (or too early) to get started.

I hope you enjoy reading this book and find inspiration within its pages. I pray the verses encourage you, the examples give you hope, and the recipes give you something new to try as you focus on putting nourishing foods in your body.

Your Journey to Wellness

"For I know the plans I have for you," declares the LORD, "Plans to prosper you and not to harm you, plans to give you hope and a future." (Jeremiah 29:11)

You have decided to reboot your life and begin your journey to better health. Over the past fifteen years of owning a wellness retreat and being a health counselor, I have met many people who have a goal of wellness, if not just a goal of losing weight. I myself at many times in my life have created this crazy, unattainable goal of "where I should be," not even caring about my own health and well-being or how I got there.

The first step in anyone's journey should be this: Accept yourself for where you are currently. It takes time and effort to get healthy and lose weight (if weight loss is the desired result). Begin in a good place by accepting yourself where you are and take that first step forward.

God gives us grace. Don't beat yourself up! God loves us just how we are ... flaws and all. We know God gave us this incredible instrument called our human body. There are 37.2 trillion cells in our body, and God loves every one. He even knows the number of hairs on our heads. God knows that we make mistakes, and when we ask, we are forgiven, but the extra pounds from an unhealthy diet and the wrinkles from years of unprotected sun exposure do not just vanish overnight. It takes work.

We are where we are because of the mistakes we have made, the unhealthy patterns we have developed over our lifetime and, in some cases, were even raised with. However, God still has a plan for us, and His will reigns supreme! We can have hope in our future because He has a plan to prosper us. Isn't that amazing? What an awesome thought that God is in our corner.

It could even be God's plan for you to help others either on your journey to wellness or through a new career in this growing industry. You could be thinking, "What? I'm sitting here with a belly roll hanging over my waistband!" But you know what? God can use that.

Keep in mind:

Nutrition is key: If you think you can shed pounds simply by mustering up the willpower to make up for the extra calories with exercise, chances are you won't get as far as you'd like. Exercise has numerous benefits, but weight loss is limited. What you eat and how much is far more important to weight loss.

Diets don't work: If you are wanting to lose weight just so you can look a certain way, you are setting yourself up to fail, because the weight will come back. That's the conclusion of one researcher, Traci Mann, who studied diets for twenty years at the University of Minnesota's Health and Eating Lab. When you are operating at a calorie deficit, your body is starving, and processes kick in to make you hungrier so that you seek more calories. That's a lot of willpower to overcome. A better goal, says Ms. Mann, is to know what your body's healthy weight range is and aim toward the lower end of that range. You will have a much easier time maintaining this weight, and you'll be healthier.

Acknowledge: We all know it's easy for guilt and shame to settle in when we contemplate our failures. Perhaps you were once slim, strong, and attractive back in your teens and twenties, and you feel badly because you didn't take time to maintain your weight and your health. Or perhaps you've had a tendency to blame outside factors: your job, your schedule, your spouse, or the poor eating habits your parents taught you. Neither gives you a great start to losing weight.

You can't be comfortable in your skin until you know who you are and are willing to open up and admit it. I've never met anyone who didn't have weaknesses. But I've met a lot of people who have blind spots. They won't acknowledge or admit where they fall short.

To begin, admit where you have fallen short. A simple, straightforward admission can be empowering. And there are other things to gain: insight on your triggers, along with a sense of ownership and control as you take the first step in reclaiming your health.

Attitude is important: Again, stay away from the "diet" mind-set. A better approach is to reframe your mission. Tell yourself you are getting healthy. Tell yourself you're going to spend some time detoxifying. Tell yourself you're going to re-train your brain to crave nutritious whole foods instead of salt, sugar, and fried foods. Tell yourself you are going to make better choices going forward, learning to see opportunities to find and select good, nutrient-dense foods. Put a note to remind yourself on the refrigerator!

Prayer: Starting today, constantly check in with your body while you eat, and pray for God to give you strength to only put healthy foods in small quantities in your mouth. Make basic observations about the food, how it smells, how it tastes, how you like the texture, how your body and emotions are responding to it. In studies by Lilian Cheung, a nutritionist at the Harvard School of Public Health, people who paid attention to their food intake maintained their weight loss longer than those in the control group.

Change your setting: The April 2015 issue of *Experience Life* magazine published an article by Laurel Kallenbach titled

"Habit-Changing Vacations" that proved vacation is an ideal time to replace a bad habit with a good one. The article focused on four different vacation-goers in different parts of the country seeking to change a habit. One of the subjects was a guest from our wellness retreat in Vermont. The article found that when you switch settings, your daily triggers are disrupted and your old rewards are gone, leaving you time to focus on building new patterns. Take a week to get out of your normal environment and only serve yourself nutritious, low-calorie meals. Take cooking classes and learn a new exercise so you can put your new habits to work when you get home.

Cornell University's School of Hotel Administration did a study for the Destination Spa Group my husband and I had the opportunity to be involved with. The study resulted in a recommendation that businesses send their top managers on retreat-type vacations. It concluded that a vacation is the ideal time to replace a bad habit with a good one and makes people less stressed.

Put God first in your life! Not only is this important to our relationships with others and our careers, but it's also important for our health and every other facet of our lives. Remember what Philippians 4:13 says: "I can do all things through Christ who strengthens me!"

Simple Steps for Every Day

"So do not fear, for I am with you; do not be dismayed, for I am your God. I will strengthen you and help you; I will uphold you with my righteous right hand." (Isaiah 41:10)

When we have guests at our wellness retreat in Vermont, they expect to eat well and exercise. However, when individuals get home and their stress returns, many people need an outline to remind themselves how to maintain a healthy lifestyle. For you, starting this new journey of wellness might seem overwhelming, but don't be dismayed! You are being armed with the right information. Ask God for the strength to follow it. He is there to help.

My position is, if you eat good, healthy food in reasonable portions, the weight will come off if it needs to, or you will maintain your current weight—in which case, your body is already at the weight is should be. Keep in mind, God made us all different! It is very possible that you are at the weight you should be, even if you don't like the way you are shaped.

At the retreat, we only serve meals made with fresh, healthy ingredients that are free from GMOs. It is a suggested route for everyone to take. Getting good nutrients instead of empty calories, salt, and fat from processed food will make you feel satisfied and healthy.

There are simple recipes included in the back of this book. Many of these are tried-and-true after decades of use at our wellness retreat. No fad diets—just real, true recipes to nourish your body.

You don't have to eat certain foods at certain times to be doing it "right." My philosophy as a certified health coach is simply centered on the notion that eating should be delicious, joyful, and healthy. Ecclesiastes 9:7 states, "Go, eat your food with gladness." Food should give you energy, with nutrients that heal and renew your body, yet make you feel happy and satisfied—not stuffed and guilty.

Nature-made food comes packed with the good stuff—vitamins, micronutrients, minerals, and fiber—delivering the important nutrients that sustain life the way God created it.

And then there is processed food, which contains high amounts of salt, sugar, and fat. Over time, these foods alter our sense of taste, extend our waistlines, and damage our cardiovascular systems. In addition to all that, these packaged foods include many extra ingredients designed to enhance flavor and extend shelf life. But the health effects from these additives can range from questionable to inadvisable. Instead of nourishing our bodies, these ingredients feed our cravings and actually make us less healthy in the long run. Here are just a few reasons to quit your packaged-food habit:

Hydrogenated oils: On the nutrition label, regular peanut butter (hydrogenated) is somewhat comparable to natural peanut butter in some categories, such as protein, vitamins, and minerals. The difference, however, is that hydrogenated peanut butter often has trans fats, which lowers "good" cholesterol (HDL) and raises the bad cholesterol (LDL). If a label advertises zero trans fats, verify this by checking the ingredients list for hydrogenated oils. Food labeling requirements allow food makers to round down to zero for advertising purposes. So, look for natural peanut butter with a super-brief list of ingredients. All you need to see is crushed peanuts and perhaps a bit of salt and oil.

Aspartame: For many, this artificial sweetener may serve as a green light to keep chugging soda. Yes, it does spare you from sugar's empty calories, but studies show this stuff is actually counterproductive to weight loss. It alters the brain's sweet receptors and prolongs sugar cravings. Researchers also found that over a decade, diet soda drinkers had a 70 percent greater increase in waist circumference than non-diet soda drinkers.

Butylated hydroxyanisole (BHA): This preservative keeps fat from going rancid in foods like potato chips, butter spreads, processed meats, cake mixes, and more. Whether it causes cancer in humans is up for debate, but the European Union has classified this as an endocrine disruptor that can mess with your hormones. If I were in a debate about the subject, I would lean toward it causing cancer, as well as infertility, but that is my own unscientific theory.

Nitrites: In October 2015, the World Health Organization deemed processed meats such as hot dogs, bacon, and lunch meat as carcinogens that raise the risk of colon cancer. While the warning did not point to any one thing, nitrites added to red meat have been linked to cancer in animal studies. Red meat contains a type of iron that stimulates the growth of a cancer-causing compound in the gut.

Potassium sorbate: Both Dr. Jeffery Sharpiro, MD and a 2010 article in *ScienceDirect* state that in a lab study, this preservative damaged DNA in human blood cells. Further investigation will be needed to determine the true risk. If you don't want to chance it, just be aware that it can be found in things you may be consuming to boost your health, such as dried fruit, beef jerky, and dietary supplements.

Clever food engineering: Sometimes, it's a matter of construction that can mess with our perceptions and make us want to eat more. Take the cheese puff. It is built on the principle of "vanishing caloric density." The air pockets built into this tasty snack trick your brain into thinking you are not getting enough calories, so it tells you to eat more.

Instead of filling your body with fats and mysterious chemicals that may harm you in ways we don't yet understand, know what you are putting into your body. Focus on real food, whole grains, fresh, lean meat, and plant foods that come in natural packaging, the way God intended!

So now you have some information on why you should eat clean, healthy food the way God created it, but what about those days you call on God for strength because you have a constant hunger to satisfy? That is called emotional eating. Know the forces that trigger your emotional eating and how you can tame them.

There are many people who have issues with alcohol or cigarettes, and efforts to quit these habits are often met with lots of support. Friends will make sure individuals aren't tempted. People who are trying to quit smoking can easily find places to go where it is prohibited. But, what about trying to quit an emotional food addiction? It's everywhere! Your friends and loved ones offer it to you. It's at work, school, after church in the vestibule, MOPs meetings, and sporting events. There is just no getting away from the doughnut holes and coffee cake.

I remember when I was in my late twenties and had put on almost a hundred pounds. There was not a day that went by that I didn't wake up to start a new "diet." However, each day I got hungry and shaky, and of course someone had some kind of celebration at the office. So, I was left to eat a huge piece of whatever-it-was that was being given out, only to then feel like a failure—which then led me to go home feeling like I had already blown it, so I'd binge again. It was a vicious cycle.

What is your trigger? Maybe it's just a bad day. Or maybe it's just not such a great one. In any case, you are probably feeling stressed, depressed, lonely, or bored. And with that comes an intense craving for food. Something crisp and fatty, or something with so much sugar that it could be synonymous with "diabetes."

You know it's a bad idea. But food can be like a faithful friend in these low moments. It's always there for you, tasting so good and delivering a burst of needed pleasure.

Emotional eating and food addictions have a way of kicking in when stress and emotions run high. In these situations, poor eating choices become a natural response. We'll take a deeper look at how these intense cravings kick in and steps you can take to overcome them.

It's not in your head. When we compare chocolate desserts and cheese-coated corn chips to a drug, we are actually onto something. The idea that overindulging on junk food is a real addiction is gaining support in the scientific and medical world. Take this study by Yale: When a food addict sees a milkshake, the same pleasure and reward centers in the brain activate as those of a cocaine addict. In other words, the struggle is real.

Try prayer. Many places that deal with overeating and wellness use the word, "mindfulness" or the phrase "mindful eating." However, if you are going to be mindful when you eat, why not go to God in prayer? Ask Him for strength. Ask Him to bless the healthy food you are consuming and to take the cravings away. With each bite, be thankful that you have the opportunity to eat healthfully. When you want to dive in and start some binge eating, take a moment to pray. Don't judge yourself or the people you are eating with. Just ask Jesus to help you eat slowly. Acknowledge any emotions you are feeling and any sensations in your body that are coming up to make you want to make a bad choice. Do the same anytime before meals or snacks, acknowledging emotions and sensations. Over time, you will be more in control of your emotional and physical hunger.

Put the junky stuff out of reach! A great first step is to make your object of craving more difficult to access. For example, leave your cash at home so you don't raid the vending machine at work. Sure, you can always hop in the car and grab a treat at the convenience store, but if this source of junk food is more difficult to access than the vending machine, your chances of moving past that intense craving are much higher.

Build new habits to replace your old ones and set yourself up for success. For example, keep fresh fruits and cut-up veggies handy so you can easily reach for them when hunger strikes. A great way to build a new habit is to remove yourself from your daily environment for a while and use that time and space to start building new habits that reinforce a healthier way of life.

Be patient with yourself. This takes time! Did you succumb to the drive-through? Don't beat yourself up. Stay tuned in to your inner dialogue and just ask God again for strength. Berating yourself will send you into a negative spiral that will set you up, not-too-nicely, for the next intense craving. Short-circuit those bad thoughts with something more assuring and gentle—what you would tell a friend in real life, for instance.

Spend Time in Nature Exercising

Let the fields be jubilant, and everything in them; let all the trees of the forest sing for joy. (Psalm 96:12)

There is something about being in nature that heals us. Without the hum of electronics and the blue screens of our computer and phones, we can step outside and rejuvenate. It is no wonder David wrote in Psalm 23:2-3, "He makes me to lie down in green pastures; He leads me beside the still waters. He restores my soul" (NKJV). God created this for us! Take advantage of it!

These days, anxiety, depression, emotional turmoil, mood swings, and stress are common occurrences in our daily life. These things are primarily caused by our increased engagement in artificial environments and lack of time spent in nature. Research and Scriptures reveal that being outside has a miraculous soothing power that can restore our wellness. Whatever we visualize and hear has a direct connection to our mood, which affects the functioning of our glands and immune system. Nature is an immense gift that bestows us with loads of mental, physical, and emotional rejuvenation.

Being in the wellness field, it is interesting to me how industry and man can turn a simple thing like being in the outdoors that God created into something seemingly brand-new. Sure, our wellness retreat in Vermont takes people on guided hikes and we serve healthy food, but we are just the messengers providing a great service. We didn't come up with the idea, and we don't try to pretend that we did!

A few years ago, the number one trend in spa vacations was "forest bathing." I thought, *Forest bathing? People are going to take baths in the forest now?* No, it was the new term for going out in nature and walking in the forest. Hmmm ... call me crazy, but I always thought that was called "hiking," and people have been doing it for thousands of years. Really though, there isn't much to it. God created these mountains and fields and the whole beautiful earth for us to enjoy. Get out there. It will "restore your soul." It's in the Bible!

Let's say you start running, and you'd like to log five miles for the day. You have the choice to run outside on a path that winds around a lake or head to the gym and get busy on a treadmill. Which one will give you a better, longer workout? I'd bank on the lake run each and every time, due to the simple fact that you will get more exercise.

Why? It's so easy to hop off the treadmill and go home. Outdoors, however, you still have to get yourself back to your starting point by your own power, even if you slow to a walk. In the end, this serves as a good trick you can use to help you break down your goal into smaller parts. Commit yourself to the halfway or turnaround point; once there, you can focus on finishing what you've begun.

Staying away from the gym just might be a surefire way to get in shape. Here are a few more advantages to consider:

Save money on gym memberships: It goes without saying that jogging around in nature is free while running on the gym's treadmill or elliptical machine costs money. However, if you can afford it, or if your health insurance already covers the cost, then a gym membership offers a great backup plan when the weather turns foul. Otherwise, look into seasonal memberships and punch cards to see you through the worst weather.

Vitamin D: I am sure you have heard a lot of talk about the benefits of taking a vitamin D supplement—doing so can prevent cancer, lower the risk of osteoporosis, boost your immune system, and so on. However, an article in "The Nutrition Source," a publication of Harvard's School of Public Health, points out that while it is true that vitamin D is essential to health, it's difficult to obtain through your food. In fact, it's not known if supplements can deliver the benefits of vitamin D as well as the sun. You can get all the vitamin D your body needs for one week just by exposing your skin to the sun for 15 minutes. Of course, be sure you are slathering on plenty of safe, organic sunscreen for the remainder of the time you're outdoors.

More thorough, more efficient: Outside, even subtle changes to the terrain can help build leg and ankle muscles while you're running or biking. And as much as you hate biking into the wind, think of that resistance as a great workout companion—one that helps you exert more energy and build endurance.

New places, new experiences, new friends: Have you ever met anyone who wanted to ride a stationary bicycle in all fifty states? I haven't either. We do all know of someone, however, who sets out to race or bike in all fifty states. Isn't that smart? It's ambitious, it makes you healthier, and you can travel the country. Setting your sights on a scaled-back version of that plan can also be powerfully effective and rewarding. Get a map and check out some national parks, state parks, and regional trails. Then craft your own bucket list. Just be sure to wear a helmet.

It's just happier: This fact is very plain and simple: People who exercised outdoors in a natural setting came away with higher levels of satisfaction than those who had a similar workout indoors, according to a study conducted by the University of Innsbruck and reported by the Global Wellness Institute. The outdoor exercisers also reported a greater sense of well-being and had stronger intentions to repeat the activity.

Experience the difference that exerting yourself outdoors can make with regard to your strength, endurance, and state of mind. Whatever your body can handle, there is plenty for the senses, with the rich scenery, gentle nature sounds, and sweet air to serve as an antidote to a stressful life. Choosing to be outside, on a hike, is so much better than staying home and running on a treadmill. The treadmill is a great tool, but it can be a boring way to get in shape. It's hard work mustering the will to keep going. Hiking is not boring. There's no hopping off. You are in it and you must finish. Plus, you'll get a much better workout walking up and down steep inclines, along roots, logs, and rocks. Walking and hiking in a sandy area (one of my personal favorites) also increases the workout. Walking on sand actually accounts for using up to 2.7 times more energy than walking on pavement.

Exercising outside and among nature does some wonderful things for the mind and soul. Research says so. It boosts memory, and improves concentration and focus.

So, you see, you are built to benefit from the outdoors. You need this. God intended it to be that way! Even if you live in a city, finding a local park or recreation center that has an outdoor track can even give you a better boost than an indoor workout.

Nature has been referred to as vitamin "N": This vitamin lowers the level of the stress hormone cortisol in our saliva. People who live near luscious green surroundings have a lower level of this hormone than those living in a city. An outdoor walk decreases cortisol levels, sympathetic nerve activity, blood pressure, and heart rate.

Greenery beats the blues: "Nature therapy" is better than "retail therapy," as it establishes a better connection with your own body. Time in nature makes it easy to have time with God. There are no distractions other than the beauty He created. Nature is a highly rewarding and calorie-free way to uplift your mood. Whether you're having a few bad days or a tough year, staying close to nature can help even the most upset individuals.

If your brain gets blocked: Take a walk in nature. A researcher at the University of Utah, David Strayer, has stated, "We are now seeing changes in the brain and changes in the body that suggest we are physically and mentally more healthy when we are interacting with nature." Mr. Strayer and other scientists believe that nature benefits our well-being and creativity as documented by the Greater Good Science Center at UC Berkeley.

Technology versus nature: It has been seen that the creativity of people who talk on iPhones or work on laptops and tablets decreases by 50 percent in comparison to those who are engaged in activities like hiking, visiting natural landscapes, cycling, walking, or running. Hiking is an activity that is nature-based and reduces an individual's risk of disease. It improves bone density while strengthening the glutes, hamstrings, quadriceps, and the hip and lower leg muscles. Such activities offer wellness that combats stress and anxiety. They control weight while strengthening the core.

Nature restores energy, revitalizing our body and mind: The findings of public health researchers Stamantakis and Mitchell were recently reported in an article titled, "Detoxing the City Brain with Nature"—specifically that 95 percent of respondents found themselves in a peaceful state of mind after spending time outside. Their depressed, anxious, and stressed mental state turned tranquil and balanced. Furthermore, scenic photographs or posters of nature have also been known to inspire a positive mind-set and improved psychological well-being. The natural world increases concentration span and pacifies the overactive mind.

Closed or artificial surroundings are simply not what God intended for our lives: television, cell phones, tablets, laptops, and PlayStations, etc., consume a lot of our quality time. The lack of association with the natural world due to spending too much time with electronic gadgets leads to depression. I am not saying to avoid electronics at all times. They are necessary in today's world. However, we need to take breaks. My part of running the family business requires me to be on the computer a lot. I set a timer on my phone every ninety minutes to remind myself to get outside and walk for at least fifteen minutes.

Develop a habit of adding time in your daily routine to spend outdoors. This may include going for a run or walk, riding your bicycle, flying a kite, going for a swim, fishing, or gardening. It may also include time to sit in a beautiful place to quiet your thoughts and connect with God. I am always in awe of His beautiful creation!

The Truth about Your Metabolism

Behold, I will bring it health and cure, and I will cure them,
and will reveal unto them the abundance of peace and truth.
(Jeremiah 33:6 KJV)

Eating healthier food, exercising, and being in nature are three ways to increase your health and wellness. However, there may be one additional lifestyle tweak you'll need to make to get healthy and lose weight. Even if you are eating healthy food, reducing calories, and getting out for vigorous exercise, shedding pounds may still be a struggle because something may be interfering with your hormones and metabolism.

Unfortunately, modern life works against us in this regard, with our hectic schedules and chemicals that seem to be in everything. Here are several metabolism disruptors you may not be aware of. This is the truth you need to reveal healing in your life!

We already covered emotional eating and how to eat healthy. But, aside from keeping your urges in check, did you know stress may be making you fatter? Women who experience stress burn an average of 104 fewer calories than women who do not experience stress, according to a study published in *Biological Psychiatry*. God created our bodies to produce cortisol to give us energy when we're under stress. It's our body's way of anticipating a big expenditure of energy in the near future. For instance, back in the good old days, when we actually had to go out and get our food in nature, cortisol could help us flee from a predator. I'm sure you have heard of the "flight or fight" hormone. However, in today's world, we are stressing about traffic, picking up the kids from daycare on time, helping with everyone's homework and activities, and paying the mortgage. If you are a stay-at-home mom, you might stress about if you are doing enough or your husband's career. If you are a homeschool mom, add another level on top of it all. All this stress each day gives us elevated cortisol over the long term and consistently produces glucose, leading to increased blood sugar levels. In theory, you could be looking at an extra eleven pounds a year, just from feeling stressed-out all the time.

Chemicals are everywhere. Whether you drink bottled water or open a can of beans to make a quick pot of chili, pay attention to the packaging. A chemical called bisphenol A (BPA) is often used to manufacture plastics and line cans to protect them from rust. Research has found, however, that BPA may have an adverse effect on your thyroid receptor. Even though the Food and Drug Administration says it is safe, scientists don't yet know its full health effects. Also, other chemicals in food packaging, called *obesogens*, have been known to disrupt our hormones too. Consuming these can make us feel hungry when we are actually full, in addition to kicking up our fat storage rates.

Your skin is your body's largest organ, and there are many products designed to make us feel better about the skin we're in, whether we want to conceal blemishes or disguise our real age. Unfortunately, some of these products have substances that soak in, going further than skin-deep. For example, lotions and beauty products contain substances called phthalates and parabens, which are potential endocrine disruptors. Their effects on our health are not fully known or understood, so why risk it?

Take steps to make sure your metabolism is running optimally. Control your stress with prayer and nature breaks and other relaxation techniques, such as a massage. Choose foods that come in boxes or in their fresh, whole form, and look for skin care products from a reputable health store that puts a premium on natural ingredients.

You can exercise and eat healthy food all day, every day, but it won't help if you are sabotaging yourself with chemicals from every direction. We will cover this more in other chapters.

Benefits of Massage and Bodywork

"They will place their hands on sick people, and they will get well." (Mark 16:18)

Massage treatment is the scientific and systematic treatment of the soft tissues in the body. Massage treatments are performed to achieve and maintain the conditions of a healthy body. It is among the oldest professions known to humankind. Massage treatment has been used for many years to ease muscle stress and reduce pain. It has been utilized by many societies as a healing tool. Touching is a purely natural tool for imparting support and compassion, and it is also a natural human response to pain.

When you hit your knee or bump your head, what do you do? Normally you rub it, because the rubbing will help it feel better. It is an instinctive response. Throughout history, healers have developed a variety of treatment techniques that calm the muscles and help reduce pain. With time, these have been fine-tuned into the process of massage treatment and bodywork.

It amazes me how God created our bodies. Twice I have completed ten weeks of Rolfing sessions. In addition to my chronic hip pain completely subsiding, many times I felt as though God was helping me get rid of things I was carrying around emotionally. I once heard the saying "you can carry your issues in your tissues." Just as I believe God sends us doctors to prescribe the right medicine, I believe God can send us a good bodyworker to help ease the pain in our bodies without medication. Whether you go to a chiropractor, certified massage therapist, or someone who specializes in structural bodywork (Rolfing), the results can be amazing.

Getting Rolfing often arouses emotional responses in bodies that can be mild and practically unnoticeable or strong and cathartic. It provides changes in the body through various neurobiological mechanisms that affect the functioning of the brain, having a particular impact on the regions associated with emotions and feelings. The result is that people who have gotten bodywork often report feeling more stable.

Research by Dr. Antonio Damasio, professor of neuroscience and director of the Brain and Creativity Institute of the University of Southern California, indicates that body states (with regard to the chemical, visceral, and musculoskeletal) are key factors in the formation of what we call feelings. Because good bodywork can make such profound changes to the musculoskeletal system, it is no wonder that changes in emotional states often result.

Let's face it, we have all had people who have mistreated us and we've all experienced unfair situations. God doesn't want us to carry all that weight and baggage with us. We should hand it over to Him. He alone can restore us and will make right what is wrong, but He also sends people to help us get through this. I personally found a lot of help in Rolfing, and I highly recommend it for a complete wellness lifestyle.

It was during my sessions of Rolfing and massage that I experienced deep forgiveness. We all have had people that have "done us wrong," and I am no exception. I used my quiet time on the table to reflect on my life and to pray for the emotional healing that I needed. On one day in particular, I was experiencing deep massage in my neck region, and a memory came back to me of a day when I was choked by someone very close to me. I had completely forgotten about the incident, however, I had a long, deep-seated resentment for this person. The person was no longer in my life, but the remnants of the relationship had lingered in a not-so-healthy way. It was during this hour that the memory came rushing back (remember: the issues are in your tissues), and I prayed to God that I would be able to forgive that person.

Forgiveness came and a burden was lifted. I don't believe the memory would have come up if I hadn't experienced the bodywork in that area of my neck. I prayed right there on the massage table for God to heal those long-festered wounds. My prayers were answered, and to this day, I look at people who intentionally do wrong to others with compassion. For these people are acting out to others how they feel about themselves. I am now able to recall memories of this person with compassion instead of hatred; after all, for someone to act that way toward another, it must be because they are reacting to their own set of horrible circumstances. It was emotional healing I experienced on that day, and I believe God led me to this particular bodywork therapist to have my neck area worked on. Not only were tightened muscles released, but so was a memory that had been locked away.

In addition to the mental benefits of massage, it also improves circulation and allows the body system to pump oxygen and essential nutrients into tissues. Massage even energizes the lymph flow, the body's defense system against harmful invaders. For instance, in breast cancer sufferers, massage has been proven to boost the cells that help battle cancer.

Massage increases blood circulation and lymph systems that boost the condition of the body's biggest organ: the skin. It also soothes and softens damaged and overused muscles, decreases spasms and aches, and increases joint versatility. Massage reduces healing time, helps prepare for intense workouts, and reduces subsequent aches and pains in athletes at any stage.

Massage increases range of movement and reduces distress for patients with back pain. It also provides exercise and stretching for muscles and will reduce restricting of the muscles for people with a limited range of motion.

Receiving massage regularly is more helpful than you might think. Most people may argue that you do not need regular massage and bodywork therapies. This could not be further from the truth. Regular and frequent massage treatments can play a huge part in how strong you feel now and later on. Massage treatments must be a constant part of your overall healthcare program. It may feel as if you are pampering yourself, but keep in mind that massage is beneficial.

In my thirties I dealt with incredible hip pain. I had been to many doctors to no avail. I actually had begun to walk with a limp because the pain was so bad. It radiated down my leg and often was so debilitating in the morning that I almost couldn't walk. However, after twenty weeks of once-a-week massage/body treatments with a therapist who massaged the hip muscles and the surrounding area that included my leg and feet, the pain completely went away. You might be wondering why the feet would affect my hip, but working on your feet (the foundation of how you stand) helped even out my gait, and eventually the pain went away. I received those sessions six years ago, and the pain has not returned.

Massage therapists and bodyworkers need to be researched beforehand. Ask them questions and find out their beliefs. There is a trend today in the spa industry for massage and bodywork to be very "New Age" focused. Be sure to look online for Christian massage therapists or go to your local Christian Chamber of Commerce (available in larger cities) to find one they recommend.

Benefits of Quiet Time

"But when you pray, go into your room, close the door and pray to your Father, who is unseen. Then your Father, who sees what is done in secret, will reward you."
(Matthew 6:6)

One of my favorite hymns goes:

> I come to the garden alone,
> While the dew is still on the roses,
> And the voice I hear falling on my ear,
> The Son of God discloses.

I can picture my mother singing it in church with the beautiful stained-glass windows in the background. It's one of my favorite memories.

As a busy mom who homeschools and tries to work from home running a business, I can tell you that I need my quiet time! When I don't get my quiet time, and my one-on-one prayer time with Jesus and devotions in silence, I don't recharge my batteries like I need to. And, if I am able to do all of the above, in the morning, with a cup of coffee, before everyone else in the house wakes up ... I know it's going to be a good day!

Everyone has quiet times to enjoy if we wish to. In the middle of busy lives and hectic demands, we can take little rests and enjoy relaxing moments with God. However, you can miss these moments if you are distracted by looking at your social media account or spending your time chatting on your cell phone. To really benefit from these moments, you have to become more conscious of them and connect with God. When waiting for your child to come out of school, you could spend that time worrying about your schedule, or you could enjoy a quiet moment and pray for God to take your worries and anxiety away. You will benefit from these times to calm and still your mind. These are the moments when intuition comes alive and soft whispers of motivation can bless your life.

You can find peace in simple actions like walking in a park or browsing a plant nursery. Even spending some time sitting in your yard can give you precious time to rejuvenate. Focus on the experience of God, the shades in nature, the cloud formations, and the fragrances of plants, animals, and birds. Becoming aware of God's beauty and the ambiance of the world He created, you can develop a restful outlook and a pleased heart. It is essential to build some quiet moments into one's daily plans. Quiet time will help the body relax and lower blood pressure levels and heart rate. It will allow the mind to find joy and creativity.

There are several ways to get quiet time—even ten minutes a day—when you can relax, maybe close your eyes, and talk to God about the things you are thankful for. This will allow the mind to calm and free itself from the stress of duties, which is vital to having a body that works at its best. Changing your surroundings for a short time every day can do wonders for your peace, happiness, and joy. Even if it is just leaving the living room where all the hustle and bustle of your family is or leaving the sea of cubicles at the office just to go into another room for a break can help. Just shutting out the outside world and allowing your mind and body to feel relaxed and calm. Quiet time provides better solutions to your problems, a more innovative way to complete activities, and just gives your inner self time to regroup.

Even if it is only for a few minutes every single day, it is far better than nothing. Once you have formed the practice of taking ten to twenty minutes once a day to relax and pray, you will be impressed with the energy you create when it is time to go back into the fray. Giving yourself enough time to enjoy calmness every day is more crucial than you may think.

Quiet boosts your immune system and is even essential for mental strength and conditioning. Those who pray frequently are proven to have lowered hypertension, reduced heart rates, and high quality interactions in life. The direct effect quiet has on health is amazing. For a lifestyle of total wellness, it is worth it to add a few moments of peaceful quiet into your daily life—using that time to just be with God, rest your body, and rejuvenate can give us a boost to help you get through the rest of the day.

Benefits of Fasting

"When you fast, do not look somber as the hypocrites do, for they disfigure their faces to show others they are fasting ... But when you fast, put oil on your head and wash your face, so that it will not be obvious to others that you are fasting, but only to your Father, who is unseen; and your Father, who sees what is done in secret, will reward you."
(Matthew 6:16,17–18)

Fasting. I have done it for many reasons. During my unhealthy dieting years, I often fasted just to lose weight quickly. (Note: It always came back on, plus a few more pounds.) I have fasted for medical reasons, either detoxing or for some type of medical test. I have also fasted during times when I had to make a huge life decision and was seeking clarity and answers from God.

Whatever the reason, if done correctly, the benefits associated with fasting are manifold. Mainly, we give the body a break. If you have decided to go on a meat-free fast, for instance, you may feel less bloated and heavy than normal. By fasting for designated hours, we give ourselves an opportunity to abandon the urge to consume and take a step back to examine our life a little bit more slowly. Fasting has become very popular over the years, particularly within the wellness industry, but it must be done in a healthy way and for the right reasons (not to lose inches and weight quickly). There are amazing advantages to fasting when the technique is used properly.

However, remember that maintaining a healthy diet before and after a fast is essential. Adopting a disciplined diet before the fast should be your first step. Prepare your body by completely cutting out all fast food and processed food and simply eat clean for five days prior to fasting.

Listed below are some benefits of fasting.

Fasting increases insulin sensitivity: Fasting has proven to have a good impact on insulin sensitivity, helping individuals tolerate carbohydrates in food much better than if they hadn't fasted. Research has shown that after fasting, insulin becomes more efficient at signaling cells to remove glucose from the bloodstream. When insulin levels are up, individuals have a better chance of avoiding illnesses like cancer, diabetes, and heart problems.

Fasting improves eating patterns: Fasting can be an effective practice for people who suffer from uncontrolled eating problems, and for people who cannot create a proper eating plan due to work or other factors. With irregular fasting, going without food during the midday is okay and can help you eat at a time that fits your routine. Also, for those who want to stop binge eating, you can designate a set time to eat your daily allowance of calories in one sitting and then commit to not taking another bite till the following day.

Fasting Improves brain function: Fasting has proven to increase brain functionality by enhancing the production of a healthy protein known as brain-derived neurotrophic factor (BDNF). BDNF stimulates brain stem cells to change into new neurons and also triggers other chemicals that boost neural health. This healthy protein also protects the brain's cells from changes related to Parkinson's and Alzheimer's disease.

Fasting helps with decision-making: Fasting has helped people feel connected to God for thousands of years. Fasting during decision-making will allow you to feel better both physically and consciously. Be sure not to fast while you're trying to maintain an exercise routine. Instead, find a period of time that you can have a few days to really relax, pray, fast, and seek God's will. With a light body and a clear mind, we become more aware and happy for what God has in store for us.

Fasting can help with weight reduction, but keep in mind that it should just be used to get yourself back on track with eating healthfully again. Irregular fasting will allow the body to use fat as its primary supply of energy instead of sugar. When we are in a period of back-to-back celebrations or holidays, a juice fast or watermelon fast for just a day can help us get back on track and break the cycle of binging.

Benefits of Essential Oils

"Is anyone among you sick? Let him call for the elders of the church, and let them pray over him, anointing him with oil in the name of the Lord." (James 5:14 NKJV)

Did you know that there are hundreds of verses in the Bible about essential oils? Essential oils are one of God's amazing creations and gifts. Massage therapists use them during treatments, and many people use them to scent their homes or offices. There are so many uses for these amazing oils, and they can help you on the path of wellness.

Essential oil is a concentrated and organic liquid, which is taken from the roots, stems, leaves, wood, and bark of plants. Essential oil is considered to be the oldest medicine used from nature since approximately 3500 B.C.. Maintaining a healthful life through naturopathy is gaining popularity, and aromatherapy is considered to be the art of maintaining and healing a healthy life through scent. Aromatherapy uses natural extracts such as essential oils.

Essential oil is used in aromatherapy to alleviate different health conditions, such as a cold, pain, arthritis, stress, anxiety, skin problems, and many other issues. There are several types of essential oil on the market, each with their own curative uses. As they are pure extracts, they are pricey compared to other oils. The cost of each essential oil depends on where it is grown, the scarcity of the plant, and the quality of the distiller used while extracting the oil. When inhaled, essential oils impact the olfactory receptor cells and send signals to the part of the brain generally known as the limbic system. Essential oils may also be put directly on the skin, but they should be mixed with a carrier oil beforehand.

Essential oils provide mental and physical benefits. They are good for helping people relax and can also work as a stimulant. They can even be utilized to help with anxiety, depression, and stress. Inhaling these oils is also thought to offer benefits to the lungs, and decrease congestion.

Certain essential oils not only work well on the human body but are also useful when it comes to cleaning and sanitizing the home. They are natural and do not include toxins or chemicals that may have dangerous effects. Instead, when used correctly and carefully, they can help remedy many conditions. Below is a list of essential oils and what they can be used for:

Lemon Oil & Tea Tree Oil	All-purpose cleanser
Lavender Oil	Ease anxiety
Citronella Oil & Eucalyptus Oil	Mosquito repellent
Frankincense Oil	Increased focus
Lemon Oil	Wash toxins off produce
Peppermint Oil	Detoxify the air
Cedarwood Oil	Relaxation
Chamomile	Helps with sleep
Rose Oil	Depression
Grapefruit Oil	Skin cleaner
Cedarwood Oil & Basil Oil	Itchy scalp
Ginger	Ease nausea

What an amazing gift God has given us in natural ingredients for wellness!

Benefits of Belonging to a Church Group

"That they may all be one, just as you, Father, are in me, and I in you. May they also be in us so that the world may believe that you have sent me." (John 17:21)

God intends for us to be in a church group. He wants us to feel as though we are one family. This is so important in today's fragmented society. We, as humans, thrive on being together—especially in a day and age where social media is (ironically) making people feel less connected and more lonely.

Life doesn't appear to slow down. Most people's weekdays are usually filled with work, school, extracurricular activities, cooking, and other tasks. When the weekend starts, many people just want to relax and have fun. The world is getting more secular, and going to church is not as common as it was previously. I meet so many people who consider themselves religious, yet church attendance and involvement are way down on their list of priorities. Local churches should play an important role in individuals' religious lives. They are a main source of Bible study, discipleship, worship, responsibility, support, and fellowship for Christians.

For the past fifteen years, I have (mostly) lived in Vermont half of the year and in Florida the other half of the year. Most of those years, our time in Florida was spent in Naples, but over the past few years, our time in Florida has primarily been traveling for our business. I have had the opportunity to visit so many different churches. From small country churches to mega churches, I have had the opportunity to get involved in a variety of churches during my time of traveling. I can tell you from personal experience, when you are in a new town, attending a church and getting involved is a way to feel connected. In Florida, I enjoy churches with large women's groups because I have a very social personality type. While in Vermont, I attend a church that only has about fifteen people in the congregation. While these churches are vastly different, one thing is constant: It is vitally important to be involved with other believers. It is important to feel connected and have a group of people you can rely on for prayer.

Church offers so much. God intends for us to feel like we belong and not be alone in our Christian walk. It is even important to our well-being and our health. Whether you have been a lifelong churchgoer or are new to faith, get involved. Listed below are the advantages of belonging to a church group.

Handle Pressure and Stress Better

Church groups offer great support in times of troubles and stress. You will have a sense of security and stability when you realize there are people that really care for you and are committed to stay with you. When anyone loses a job or a relative has a long-term illness or a new mother wants guidance, these are needs that require a supportive group who can come together in prayer. A church group is there for its members to help in times of need. They provide a feeling of connectedness.

Life Changes Happen in Church Groups

You may have a great personal weekend worship routine, but the best way to achieve transformation and keep progressing in the right direction is by participating in a church group. From DivorceCare, to GriefShare, to church wellness groups, life change is more apt to occur in groups at church that are made up of individuals with similar values and beliefs.

Feel Part of God's Family

Many people who have been part of a church group say there is a benefit in the friendship and close relationships that develop from worshipping together and sharing important prayer requests. Realizing that your needs and difficulties are not unique will help you recognize that other people are facing the same challenges—or have survived them and have spiritual wisdom to spare.

Deepen Your Knowledge of Worship

Just as you can't get stronger without regular workouts, you can't develop a deeper walk with God without regular worship. I have heard many people say they can have church "wherever they are." This is especially true in Vermont, which has the lowest population in the country of people who regularly attend church. However, being part of a church body gives us growth and accountability. It gives us opportunities to find belonging and Godly support—whether you are aging, have children, are newly married, or have homeschoolers.

Eliminate GMOs from Your Diet

"Or do you not know that your body is a temple of the Holy Spirit within you, whom you have from God? You are not your own, for you were bought with a price. So glorify God in your body." (I Corinthians 6:19–20 ESV)

The Bible doesn't say anything about genetically modified organisms (GMOs) because they weren't around back then. However, there is mounting evidence that they are not good for our bodies. Sometimes when I read about how damaging GMOs are to our bodies, I picture God saying, *"What have you done with My Creation?"* Let's arm ourselves with the facts. Treat your body as a temple of the Holy Spirit. Stay clear of GMOs.

GMOs include a broad selection of animals, plants, and bacteria that are made for a wide selection of applications, from agricultural manufacturing to scientific research. The kinds of possible dangers posed by GMOs differ according to the type of organism that's modified and its proposed application. Most of the problems associated with GMOs pertain to their side effects on human health and the environment. In the last few years, many countries have banned GMOs and the pesticides that go with them for a reason.

There is a lot of credible scientific research by three leading researchers at Earth Open Source that clearly shows why GMOs must not be eaten, and evidence against GMOs is growing every year. There are a number of experts around the world who oppose them. Everyone knows that GMO foods are the most controversial subjects in agriculture. Why are scientists and specialists coming forward to provide constructive feedback about GMOs in our food? Here are the amazing facts:

Reduced Nutrients

A genetically modified crop could have lower nutrients than its natural counterpart by inadvertenty eliminating some aspects of nutrition or making the nutrients indigestible. For instance, phytate (sometimes referred to as an "antinutrient") is a compound in grains and seeds that binds with nutrients and makes them impossible for humans to absorb. An inserted gene may cause a plant to create higher amounts of phytate, reducing the mineral nutrient content of that plant.

Increased Toxicity

Most plants create substances that are harmful to humans, but most of the crops that people consume produce harmful toxins at amounts low enough that they do not create any damaging effects. However, adding an exotic gene into a crop may cause it to produce harmful toxins at increased levels that could be harmful to humans—especially if other genes in the plant are destroyed during the gene insertion process, as this may cause the plant to change its natural production of toxins.

Companies selling GMOs do not want their supplies labeled, for fear of stigmatizing their products and losing buyers. Natural food companies want GMO foods labeled because they, too, suspect it will drive buyers toward their natural goods. The reason GMO food must be labeled by the food sector is that it is clear some buyers wish to know what they are consuming and they have the right to really know what is in their food. More than sixty countries require GMO labeling, including Australia, Japan and every country in the European Union. It just makes sense to know what one is putting in their body.

The opponents of labels must end their objections to allowing people to know what is in their meals. If GMO advocates and producers really thinks that GMO food is good and harmless, then they should be more than willing to add a smiley-faced DNA helix to their packaging and market out of the truth that advanced GMOs are in most of your breakfast cereals, cooking oils, soups, dairy products, and frozen foods.

Prepackaged Food Dangers

The long-term effects of artificial chemicals utilized in preserving and processing food can be damaging to human health. Small amounts of the chemical substances used in food packaging can diffuse into the food itself, and this transference can be enhanced by increased temperatures, the kind of packaging material the food is in, and the number of days the food is stored. These foods are often frozen and have to be heated in the microwave for some minutes, which is cause for even more health concerns.

Foods normally come in plastic or foam-based containers that many assume are microwave safe, but actually, most of these containers are not safe to heat and may even start to break down in the microwave. Heating unsafe packaging can release chemicals into food that cause problems such as cancer, reproductive organ damage, birth defects, and developmental problems.

These problems can affect individuals' long-term health and make them vulnerable to further illnesses and injuries. While most packaging containers are cleared before being sold as "microwave safe," that is not always the case. Also, some foods become saturated with chemicals before they are even packed. People who eat a great deal of packaged or refined foods could be chronically exposed to low amounts of these chemicals all through their lives.

A proper consumption of daily fiber is essential for the health of the digestive tract. Chronically low dietary fiber can reduce digestive system function and pave the way for opportunistic pathogens. Most refined food has little fiber and is full of processed carbohydrates. Consuming lots of fiber can protect you from heart problems and diabetes. Many refined foods are rich in taste but low in the essential nutrients that the body needs. You may be eating three full meals daily, but if those meals are mostly refined, you are likely undermining your immune and digestive systems.

Did you know that packaged meals are high in sodium? Sodium really helps add flavor to food and also helps keep food from spoiling. However, consuming a lot of sodium will cause the body to retain water, which forces your heart to operate double-time and can later result in hypertension or a serious heart disease. When you eat packaged foods, you will discover that they are fairly rich in trans fats. These fats are chemically made fats; the kind the body cannot process and can never use for any purpose. Trans fats travel around in the bloodstream, blocking the arteries and increasing cholesterol. Too much cholesterol can result in serious heart disease, or even a heart attack or stroke.

To really treat your body the way it was intended, one really does need to steer clear of GMOs and prepackaged food. When you move on to eating a clean diet full of natural food and naturally prepared foods, you will really notice a change in your body if you start eating unhealthy again. Fortunately, we are able to stock our kitchen with good, healthy foods. However, when I am traveling and find myself eating out or grabbing a quick snack at an airport (it happens), I can immediately notice the change in my body the next day. I can feel the excess water I'm retaining, and my tummy never feels right. You can train your taste buds to crave good food. Even after growing up on the food I was raised on, I can honestly tell you, I don't crave Little Debbies any longer!

Eliminating Other Toxins from Your Home and Lifestyle

"Worthy are you, our Lord and God, to receive glory and honor and power, for you created all things, and by your will they existed and were created." (Revelation 4:11 ESV)

I have mentioned that at one point in my life I had gained a hundred pounds. I often have wondered how in the world I gained so much weight. Yes, I know it was because of too much food and lack of exercise, but there was something else going on too, I am sure of it. In addition to weight gain, I also had extreme hormonal swings and the general feeling that something just was not right with my body. I went to doctors and was prescribed antidepressants and hormones; I went to counselors who gave me tips on dealing with stress; I went to a Chinese doctor who gave me a concoction of ground up herb powders; I even went to a top "weight loss" doctor in Tyson's Corner, Virginia, who gave me Fen-Phen to lose pounds. Trust me, I have been through it all when it comes to getting healthy!

It really wasn't until I married my husband and started running the business with him in Vermont that I began to realize health is not just about exercise and nutrition; it is about everything we put in our body, on our body, and around our body (what we surround ourselves with). I thank God every day that the opportunities were available for to me to get healthy and that

He sent my husband my way. I would not have learned any of this or become a health coach without God's intervention in my life.

While in Vermont, I stopped using dry cleaners (partly because I just didn't need to), I stopped getting acrylic nails, I stopped being surrounded by pesticides and chemicals, and I purposely started using more local organic products on my skin (which are plentiful in Vermont). My health and wellness improved. Hormonal imbalances were cleared up. My depression ceased. Could it all be connected? I think so. God did not intend for all these chemicals to pollute our bodies (and our minds). They are the work of man, and they are wreaking havoc on us.

Read on:

Dry Cleaning Contains Toxic Chemicals

It might seem hard to believe that the very first dry cleaning process started in France in 1845. These days, dry cleaning providers are everywhere. When people buy clothes, they do not give a thought to a "dry-clean only" label; in fact, many business clothes, uniforms, and outerwear need this kind of cleaning. But everyone should know that this kind of cleaning is dangerous because it is harmful not just to one's well-being but also to the environment (and to one's budget). Dry cleaners use tough solvents, chemicals and detergents to wash clothes. Actually, the chemicals used nowadays are all different from the chemicals that were used when dry cleaning was first introduced. Today, the hardest chemicals used are tetrachloroethylene, perchloroethylene and tetrachloroethene, known together as PERC, but there are more solvents used also.

The EPA and the International Agency for Research on Cancer have classified PERC as a toxin. A study carried out by the Environmental Protection Agency in 2012 to figure out the dangers of PERC to dry cleaners classified PERC as a "likely hu-man carcinogen." They confirmed that long-term contact with PERC increased the chance of cancers and other ailments. It is safer to wet-clean your clothes and use natural, nontoxic, eco-friendly cleaners—especially since dry cleaning chemicals can remain present in your home for up to a week. It was when I was pursuing my career in the Washington, DC, area that I experi-enced the most problems with my hormones and other feminine issues. I believe much of those problems were due to stress, but I also wore dry-clean only clothes every day. Since learning about the dangers of dry cleaning chemicals, I have not had anything on my skin that was dry cleaned for over a decade.

Toxic Pesticides and Chemicals

Pesticide-based repellents and yard treatments have become things of the past as more natural products have started to sur-face. Do you wonder how pesticides affect human lives? They may do more harm than you think to the environment, human health, and your living conditions at home.

Chemical pesticides have been related to a variety of human health risks, from temporary impacts like nausea and headaches to long-term effects like endocrine disruption and reproductive harm. Long-term health effects can occur many years after even minor contact with chemical pesticides has occurred. Adverse effects can also be triggered by the pesticide residues that we unintentionally consume through our water and food. Children are especially prone to the dangers linked to pesticide use since their nervous system, immune system, and other internal detoxi-fying mechanisms aren't fully developed, making them less ca-pable of dealing with the introduction of harmful pesticides into their bodies.

Pesticides usually contain inert substances along with ac-tive components that are made to kill the target pest. We have to make our meals, our water, our air, and our soil free from harmful chemicals. The solution to pest issues lies in nontoxic alternatives.

Potentially harmful chemicals are probably available in every space in your home. If not properly kept or used, these products may end up in the body and cause minor to severe health issues. Taking an eco-friendly approach to cleanup can help us feel better mentally, but you will also feel better physically, knowing you are developing a safer place for yourself, your household, and your pets.

While all sorts of chemical pesticides are known to infiltrate everything they come in contact with, organic products are less invasive by composition, thus reducing or eliminating recurring damage. Promoting the use of natural, food-based repellents can help get rid of harmful pesticides from the marketplace, and from the food we eat.

The Hidden Dangers in Skin Care Products

When buying skin care products, you do so with the aim of calming and pampering your skin—maybe to make it look younger or to retain its youthful glow. There is a good possibility though that the skin care products you use contain numerous potentially harmful chemicals that are of no value to the skin and can really cause harm to the body. Most of these additives are linked with endocrine disruptors.

So, what are these hidden dangers?

Parabens

Parabens are labeled as carcinogenic, which means they can cause cancer. Recent research shows that parabens can increase the chance of breast cancer in most women, in addition to

causing problems with the endocrine system. Parabens are utilized in over-the-counter shelf life of the product. These substances are found in face and body washes, body lotions, and
cleansers.

Sodium Lauryl Sulfate

This chemical is commonly used in all sorts of skin care products, from soaps to shampoos and conditioners. This is a skin
irritant that can cause eczema, dermatitis, and psoriasis. It has
been found to slow tissue treatment and can also cause cataracts.

Avoid products that contain artificial fragrances, parabens,
and mineral oils. When properly created using potent, pure ingredients, natural products are often more effective compared to
their chemically loaded counterparts.

The Benefits of a "Natural Wrapper" Diet

*And God said, "Behold, I have given you every plant yielding
seed that is on the face of all the earth, and every tree with
seed in its fruit. You shall have them for food."*
(Genesis 1:29 ESV)

T he best "fast" food comes in natural packaging. One of
the best ways to get healthy is to replace old habits with
new. Over time, those bad habits will lose their hold on
you and eventually disappear.

To help you kick your prepackaged, junk-food habit, here are
some ideas for easy snack replacements. When it's time to refuel,
don't pull into the drive-through or reach for the cheesy chips.
That processed food you crave is filled with salt, fat, and empty
calories, sapping your energy. Instead, reach for something that
comes in a natural wrapper.

Stock up on plant foods that are naturally protected and pre-
served in shells and peels. Invest a bit of time at the start of the
week to do your shopping and plan your natural wrapper snacks
and meal prep for the upcoming week. That way, when hunger
hits, you'll have easy solutions that will restore your health with
all their fiber, vitamins, minerals, and micronutrients and help
you lose weight. Every part of your body will get healthier and
thank you, including your skin, blood vessels, brain, and heart.

Oranges: In one orange, you get all the vitamin C you need for the day—and more. Plus, you get a good hit of those stress- and anxiety-reducing B vitamins, along with some heart-healthy flavonoids. Pair with a small serving of cottage cheese or Greek yogurt.

Bananas: Dieters are often discouraged from eating these tree fruits because of their relatively high calorie and carb count, but it's highly doubtful that bananas are to blame for obesity. Banan- as have lots of potassium to help your muscles recover from a workout. Plus, they have resistant starch, which keeps you feel- ing full and feeds healthy gut bacteria. Best of all, one bunch will probably cost you less than your favorite burger.

Grape tomatoes: Serving these as a snack can help you reach the seven servings a week of tomato-based foods that can help you reduce your cancer risk. Coax out a bit more beta-carotene by adding a little fat, such as olive oil.

Carrots: Loaded up with vitamin A to help your skin and mu- cus membranes repel bacteria, carrots also have vitamin K to regulate blood clotting and good bone health. To change up your snack regimen, try dipping these in a side of beet hummus.

Pea pods: Swap out those potato chips and french fries for pea pods and you'll have a low-calorie, iron-rich alternative that sup- plies plenty of satisfying crunch. Toss these into your backpack with some honey-roasted peanuts for a refreshing, reenergizing break.

Pears: This fruit is a heavy lifter in weight-loss plans because it's loaded with fiber. Eat with a small handful of almonds. Or halve the fruit, scoop out the seeds, and add a dollop of low fat or skim ricotta cheese sprinkled with cinnamon or nutmeg.

Grapes: This sweet fruit might be a great ally in your battle of the bulge: A 2015 study in the *Journal of Obesity*, suggests eating grapes can lower the risk of obesity. Pack these with some seeds, nuts, and cubes of cheese for a different spin on trail mix.

Blueberries: These little berries are packed with manganese, which helps you convert fat and protein into energy and aids in the formation of collagen. And these are just two superpowers wielded by this superfood. Turn these into a sweet frozen treat by dipping them in Greek yogurt, placing them on a baking sheet lined with parchment paper, freezing for a few hours, and then placing in a resealable plastic bag.

Peanuts: A handful of these will keep you satisfied and help you avoid extra, empty calories throughout the day. Harvard researchers found that people had an easier time sticking to a healthy eating plan when they included peanuts and peanut butter. In addition, they lived longer lives.

Favorite brand: Ezekiel bread. What could be better than bread with a Bible verse on it? I know, this chapter is about "natural wrappers," so why am I telling you to buy bread from a store? Because this is real life and not everyone has time to bake their own bread. Ezekiel 4:9 bread, frequently referred to as just Ezekiel bread, is a brand of sprouted grain bread made by Food For Life. The bread gets its name from and is based on the literal Old Testament Bible verse Ezekiel 4:9: "Take thou also unto thee wheat, and barley, and beans, and lentiles, and millet, and spelt, and put them into one vessel" (KJV). The six grains and legumes listed in the verse make up the ingredients of Ezekiel bread. Compared with regular grain, sprouted grain is lower in starch and has higher amounts of protein, minerals, vitamins (B2, B5, B6, and C), and other nutrients. Ezekiel bread claims to be a complete source of protein. We serve this to our guests in Vermont, and I serve it to my children at home. I love this bread! I've come a long way since my Wonder Bread days!

As you can see, great things come in small, natural packages. Always be on the lookout for foods that come in natural packaging, and over time, you'll feel and see the difference it makes in your life.

Make a Healthy Lifestyle Your Hobby

Finally, brothers and sisters, whatever is true, whatever is noble, whatever is right, whatever is pure, whatever is lovely, whatever is admirable—if anything is excellent or praiseworthy—think about such things.
(Philippians 4:8)

Find your passion in a healthy lifestyle. God tells us to concentrate on the things that are good and pure, so what better thing to concentrate on than a healthy lifestyle? It is an honor to God. You don't have to be perfect. We are all made of different shapes and sizes, and I can tell you that even though I have lost the weight, worked hard at keeping it off, and do healthy activities every day, I don't look the same size as when I was in modeling and pageants—but I AM healthier!

Do you have to be a size 8 to inspire others? No! We are not all meant to look a certain way. That emphasis on an ideal appearance is the media telling us a lie and making us feel as though we are not good enough. The truth is that we are children of God, and we are blessed with whatever shape He gave us! However, He does expect us to take care of it, and it is easier to do so when it is your hobby.

Rather than take up a hobby that clutters your house and drains your bank account, why not choose a hobby that renews you? A healthy lifestyle is the perfect hobby—it can make you stronger, fitter, and extend your life, adding energy and enjoyment to your work and play.

The reason diets and New Year's resolutions don't work is because people treat a healthy lifestyle as a chore. Instead, take control of your health from that center of passion and fun, and motivation will be less of a problem. Here are a few strategies and ideas to build that healthy hobby and keep the fire burning.

Cultivate what you already love to do: This is the first rule in any healthy lifestyle. If you want to boost your cardiovascular activities but loathe running, choose an alternative that you actually enjoy and make it the centerpiece to your physical activity. If hiking, swimming, or bicycling are more appealing to you, embrace it.

Invest in yourself on vacation: When you view your vacation time through this lens, possibilities open up. You might choose a summer vacation at a health and wellness resort where you can immerse yourself in healthy living with hiking, eating nutritious food, and building new friendships with fellow travelers who also desire a healthy jump-start in their lives. For shorter vacations, look at multi-day bike rides and weekend retreats. If you choose these events in fun, beautiful places you want to visit, it will be less of a chore and more of something to look forward to. In addition to that, there's the novelty aspect. New experiences stimulate learning, which will reinforce your new habits and give you a nice push ahead.

Be social: You already know that if you schedule a workout with a friend, you are more likely to show up and push yourself to complete a good workout. So, you can see how joining a community and being around others who enjoy what you do can add a special ingredient to your healthy hobby. Whatever you want to build in your life, find a friend. Enroll in a cooking class or sign up for a running club.

Give back: A great way to stay excited about your healthy hobbies is to teach others and pass the torch to newcomers. Local organizations are always looking for coaches in youth sports, so if baseball, wrestling, volleyball, or some other sport is your thing, think about volunteering. Not everyone you meet is going to catch the fire, but you'll come across a few who will make your efforts worthwhile. Perhaps organize a walking club or exercise club at church. Make exercise and devotions a weekly morning activity!

Look for "power" boosters: Interests and activities that complement your healthy lifestyle will keep you engaged and excited. Take up gardening to feed your interest in healthy food with fresh veggies. Take a weekend class in scenic photography and you'll add a new challenge to your weekend hikes or power walks!

Surround Yourself with Good People

Do not be deceived: "Bad company ruins good morals."
(1 Corinthians 15:33 ESV)

Whoever walks with the wise becomes wise, but the companion of fools will suffer harm. (Proverbs 13:20 ESV)
God does not mean for us to have toxic people in our lives. We can love them and show them the love of Christ by being kind to them. However, sometimes that means loving someone and praying for them from afar. Toxic relationships are not good for us physically or emotionally.

Before you make a major life change, such as getting healthy and focusing on wellness, be mindful of the one thing that can make all the difference. I'm not talking about hiring an expensive private trainer. I'm not talking about sipping on ten-dollar specialty smoothies with organic kale and chia seeds (although they are great!).

I'm talking about the people in your life. Before you embark on the winning path, it's important to take account of the people who surround you. Family, friends, colleagues—if they are having a positive impact in your life, that's an important ingredient in your journey toward change. Their positive words will give you fuel to move forward. On the other hand, people who carry bad energy and bring you down can put a drag on your momentum in ways you may not be aware of.

First, consider the traits of a good friend and a toxic friend.

A good friend is someone who is supportive. They encourage you and give you credit even when you flounder. They celebrate victories even when you are not around and encourage your walk with God. A good friend has integrity and follows through on promises. They will offer a hand, their resources, or a listening ear when you need it.

On the other hand, a toxic friend has conditions on the relationship. Without tangible things that bring an advantage to their lives, whether that's money, skills, or your willingness to babysit for free, there would be no relationship. They are unavailable physically and emotionally when you need them. Lastly, they are a bad influence and ignore your efforts to change your life. They might even try to tempt you.

Make no mistake, none of us is perfect. Keeping this in mind, be aware that the people who surround you have strengths and weaknesses. Even the good people in our lives are going to throw obstacles in our path toward winning. So, think ahead. If there are obstacles in your way to reducing contact with a toxic person, can you find ways to neutralize the bad effects of the relationship?

Sometimes there are people you do just need to cease having contact with. People who are emotionally or physically abusive, in many cases, need to exit your life. I understand how hard it can be to cut ties with relatives or those who may live under the same roof as you; however, someone who negatively affects your health is not meant to be in your life. Not every relationship is meant to last. Of course it's difficult to walk away from a sibling, a cousin, or someone else you grew up with from birth, but concluding hurtful relationships is necessary in order to go on and live a healthy, happy, whole life. You can always love and pray for someone from afar, but you need to keep dysfunction out of your life.

Be a Friend to You

Finally, consider the most important friend of all on this earth. You have probably neglected this friend for a long time. Starting today, make a true effort to like this person and speak with kind words to them. We're talking about you. God loves you. You are special. Be kind to yourself!

It sounds corny, but think about it. What do you say to a friend when she stumbles in her efforts to quit smoking? Do you call her a stupid, ugly failure? If she goes off track with her healthy eating plan by downing a pint of ice cream, do you tell her she just isn't cut out for the challenge? Of course not. Why do you let yourself get away with making these awful statements to yourself? These statements set yourself up to fail. Say positive things to yourself and pray constantly for God to help you through the day.

Think about what you value most in a friend and look for opportunities to be that friend. When you promise yourself you're going to go running, follow through. When you are having a bad day, say something nice to yourself. Kindness will give you a lift and the momentum to succeed. Change, after all, starts from the inside. Your relationship with yourself is a good place to start.

Target Your Habits for Lasting Wellness

"In the morning, O LORD, You will hear my voice; in the morning, I will order my prayer to You and eagerly watch."
(Psalm 5:3 NASB)

S tart new habits and pray for strength and guidance before your feet even hit the floor each morning. Eagerly watch what God is doing in your life. He has good plans for you! You may have heard this saying: Good habits are hard to form but easy to live with. On the flip side of that, however, are bad habits. For instance, it was easy enough finishing off those bags of chips, bowls of ice cream, and plates of homemade mac and cheese topped with pulled pork. But today, it's hard to live with the results. Doing the good stuff is hard. If it were easy, everyone would eat healthy.

At the core of eating healthy and living a life geared toward wellness is targeting your habits.

Anatomy of a Habit

Triggers: Even when we begin our day with willpower set to maximum intensity, our brains are hardwired to look for simple solutions that feel good when we are stressed. When stress occurs, it's in our DNA to crave more calories and rest. This served our species well back when resources were scarce and we needed to conserve energy. But it's not helpful when you have a huge deadline and there is a bag of chips in your line of vision.

Routine: Up to 40 percent of the time, your actions are not driven by decisions; they are driven by habit, according to research. We do things all day long we don't even think about. So when we are triggered, certain actions kick in.

Rewards: When you take that first bite of whatever it is you crave, that's the payoff. It doesn't matter if you feel guilty, because that reward system that floods your brain with pleasure-filled dopamine is much more powerful. By the way, one study has shown that eating a lot of fatty food can slowly change your brain's reward circuit; over time, you will need to add more of it to get the same hit of pleasure.

Anatomy of Lasting Change

To make your healthy new habits stick, here is what the research tells us works best:

Identify your cycles: Instead of thinking about the overall goal of eating healthy to achieve a healthy weight, look for key moments throughout the day when you stumble and end up eating what you shouldn't. Make a list. Be honest. Those are the cycles you want to break and overthrow.

Replace the habit: Self-discipline is a limited resource in a day, and stress is taxing to it, according to Jenny Evans, an author, speaker, and expert on resiliency and stress. Know what your triggers are and keep easy solutions ready and within reach. For example, if you want to kick the fast-food habit at work, keep a stockpile of nutritious food that tastes good to you. Is it doughnut day at work? Keep a pack of gum in your desk and pop a stick in your mouth when you crave that cream-filled, chocolate-covered sugar bomb of fat and simple carbs. If nighttime snacking is your downfall, spend part of your Saturday evening cutting crisp, fresh veggies you like so you'll have a ready snack that's just as convenient as the bag of chips you're longing to devour.

Have a plan: You may wake up one day to discover your old eating habits have crept back into your life. If you fail, you can bounce back. First, get ahead of it. Make a relapse plan when those pounds start creeping upward, and set your maximum weight that will trigger you to take action. When you hit that upper weight, implement your plan and tighten the controls that helped you shed pounds in the first place.

To overthrow your bad habits, make a few changes to your environment. During your time in prayer and devotions, figure out what is triggering your habits and what you can do to stop the cycle. It's hard, but setting yourself up for success means that you can eventually find it.

May God bless you on your journey of wellness! Seek Him first and follow His guidance. I hope this book helps you on your path. In the meantime, healthy and natural food recipes that we have used at our wellness retreat for many years are listed for your use.

Be well.

In Christ,

Kathleen LeSage

Recipes

BREAKFAST RECIPES

Blender Breakfast Drink
1/4 cup yogurt
1 cup apple juice or milk
1 banana
2 tsp wheat germ
1 tbsp molasses or honey (or to taste)
6 almonds
1 tsp yeast powder (optional)
2 tsp protein powder (optional)
Blend all ingredients in a blender until smooth. Serves 1.
• Instead of banana, use 8 strawberries; a quarter cantaloupe or honeydew melon; or 1 apple, peach or nectarine.
• This is a good quick breakfast that's easy to make, very filling, low in fat, and an overall great way to start the day off right.

Honey Banana Bread
2 cups whole wheat pastry flour
1/2 cup whole cane sugar or brown sugar
1 tsp baking powder
1 tsp baking soda
2 tsp cinnamon
1/2 tsp nutmeg and salt (optional)
1 tsp vanilla

3 ripe bananas, mashed
2 eggs
3 tsp plain or vanilla yogurt
Spritzed oil
Preheat oven to 350°F. Mix dry ingredients in a large bowl and then add wet ingredients, mixing well to combine. Spritz a 9 × 5-inch loaf pan with oil. Spread batter into pan and bake for 45–50 minutes, or until toothpick inserted into center comes out clean. Remove from oven and let stand for 10 minutes. Invert onto a wire rack or serving board and slice once completely cool.
• Walnuts, raisins, and dried cranberries all make wonderful additions to this recipe. Add about 1/3 cup of your choice.

Mushroom Omelet
Spritzed oil
2 cups freshly sliced mushrooms
1/4 tsp tamari
3 eggs, beaten
Spritz a skillet with oil and sauté mushrooms over medium heat, then add tamari. Spritz a separate omelet pan with oil, add eggs, and cook over medium heat until bottoms of eggs are solid. Add mushrooms. Fold eggs over mushrooms. Cook additional 1–2 minutes.

Oatmeal Pancakes
1/2 cup whole wheat flour
1 1/2 cups rolled oats
1 1/2 cups milk
1 egg
2 tsp molasses
3 tsp baking powder
Spritzed oil
Pure maple syrup

Mix dry ingredients in a large bowl and wet ingredients in a separate, smaller bowl. Pour wet ingredients into dry ingredients and stir until blended. Spritz a skillet or griddle with oil over medumhigh heat. Ladle batter onto griddle and cook pancakes on for approximately 3 minutes on each side. Top with pure maple syrup. Serves 2.

Cinnamon Raisin French Toast
8 slices cinnamon raisin bread
4 eggs
1/3 cup milk
1/2 tsp nutmeg (optional)
1/8 tsp allspice (optional)
Spritzed oil
Pure maple syrup
Beat together eggs, milk, and spices. Dip bread in egg mixture, coating both sides. Spritz a skillet or griddle with oil over medium-high heat, then cook bread slices for 3 minutes on each side or to desired doneness. Top with pure maple syrup. Serves 4.

SOUPS & SALAD RECIPES

Yummy Avocado Dressing
1 avocado, pitted and peeled
1 garlic clove, peeled
1/4 cup cilantro
1 tbsp fresh lime juice
2 tbsp avocado oil or olive oil
1/4 tsp sea salt
In a blender or food processor, add all ingredients and blend until smooth. To thin the dressing, add up to a half cup water until

it is the consistency you desire. You can keep it in the fridge for a day or so, but it always tastes best freshly made. (That's how we serve it to our guests in Vermont!)

Kale & White Bean Soup
1 tbsp olive oil
1/2 small onion, chopped
1 small bunch kale, stemmed and coarsely chopped
1 (14.5-oz) can cannellini (white kidney) beans, drained
4 cups low-sodium chicken broth
Sea salt and freshly ground black pepper (to taste)
Heat oil in a large, heavy-bottomed pot over medium heat. Add onion and garlic and cook, stirring occasionally, until onion is soft (6–8 minutes). Add kale and continue cooking, tossing occasionally, until wilted (about 3 minutes). Add beans and broth and bring to a boil. Reduce heat and simmer 15–20 minutes; season with salt and pepper. Divide soup among bowls. 4 servings.

Coconut Carrot Soup
1/4 cup (1/2 stick) unsalted butter
1 lb carrots, peeled and chopped
1 medium onion, chopped
Sea salt and freshly ground black pepper (to taste)
2 cups low-sodium chicken broth
1 (5-oz) can unsweetened coconut milk
2 tbsp Thai-style chili sauce
Fresh cilantro leaves (for garnish)
Melt butter in a large saucepan over medium-high heat. Add carrots and onion, season with salt and pepper, and cook, stirring often, until carrots are softened (15–20 minutes). Stir in broth, coconut milk, and chili sauce. Bring to a boil, then reduce heat and simmer, stirring occasionally, until vegetables are very soft and liquid is slightly reduced (40–45 minutes). Let soup cool slightly, then purée in a blender until smooth. Reheat in a

saucepan, thinning with water to desired consistency and sea-soning with salt and pepper. Divide soup among bowls and top with cilantro. 4 servings.

Curried Butternut Squash Soup
1/4 cup unsweetened coconut flakes
1/4 cup pumpkin seeds
1 large butternut squash (about 3 lb), peeled, halved lengthwise, and cut into 3/4-inch slices
1 small onion, quartered
4 garlic cloves, peeled
1/4 cup plus 1 tbsp virgin coconut oil, melted
3 tbsp curry powder
Sea salt and freshly ground black pepper (to taste)
1/3 cup cilantro, chopped
2 tsp finely grated orange zest
1 1/2 cups coconut milk
2 cups hot water
Preheat oven to 350°F. Toast coconut flakes on a rimmed baking sheet, tossing occasionally, until golden brown (3–5 minutes); transfer to a small bowl. Toast pumpkin seeds on baking sheet, tossing occasionally, until golden brown (4–6 minutes). Let cool slightly, coarsely chop, and add to bowl with coconut flakes; set aside.
Increase oven temperature to 450°F. Toss squash, onion, garlic, oil, and curry in a large bowl until squash is coated; season with salt and pepper. Arrange in a single layer on baking sheet and roast, turning occasionally, until squash and onion are browned and tender (40–50 minutes).
Meanwhile, add cilantro and orange zest to reserved coconut flakes and pumpkin seeds and stir to combine. Season with salt and pepper and cover.
Purée garlic, squash, onion, curry, coconut milk, and hot water in a blender until smooth, adding more water if needed. Season

with salt and pepper. Serve soup topped with coconut flake mixture. 4–6 servings.

Cucumber Papaya Poppy Seed Salad

2 cucumbers, peeled or unpeeled (according to preference), seeded and chopped
1/2 cup diced dried papaya
1/4 cup nonfat plain yogurt
Juice of 1 lemon
1 tsp poppy seeds
1 tsp Dijon mustard
1 tbsp freshly chopped parsley
1 garlic clove, chopped
Coarsely ground black pepper (to taste)
Place all ingredients in a bowl, mix well, let sit for a half hour in the refidgerator, and enjoy!

Black Bean Soup

2 cups dry black beans, or 3–4 (15-oz) cans rinsed and drained black beans
1 strip kombu seaweed (optional)
1 large onion, diced
4 garlic cloves, minced
3 tsp olive oil
2 tsp cumin
2 tsp chili powder
2 tsp coriander
3 celery stalks, diced
2 medium carrots, diced
2 fresh tomatoes or 1 (6-oz) can tomato paste
2 tsp basil
2 tsp oregano
2 tsp no-salt vegetable broth
Freshly ground black pepper (if desired, to taste)

Tamari (if desired, to taste)
Yogurt (for garnish)
Chopped scallions (for garnish)
If desired, soak dry beans in water for several hours prior to cooking and discard water. Simmer beans for 2 hours in 8 cups water (or 6 cups if beans are presoaked) and kombu, if desired. In a separate pan, heat oil over medium heat and sauté onion, garlic, cumin, chili powder, and coriander until onion is translucent. Add celery and carrot and continue cooking for 15 minutes. Add tomatoes, basil, oregano, broth, and sautéed vegetables to cooked black beans and simmer for 30 minutes. Garnish with yogurt and chopped scallions. Serves 6.

Mushroom Soup
Spritzed oil
1 large onion, chopped
1 lb fresh mushrooms, sliced
1/4 cup tamari
1 tsp ground black pepper
1 qt water
2 tbsp freshly chopped chives
Spritz a 2-quart pot with oil over medium heat. Add onions and sauté until clear. Add mushrooms and continue to sauté until mushrooms are browned. Add tamari and pepper, stirring to mix. Add water and heat just to boiling point. Add chives. Serve immediately. Serves 4–6.

Onion Soup
6 medium onions, sliced
1/4 cup tamari, divided
Spritzed oil
1 quart water
2 tablespoons sherry
Ground black pepper (to taste)

1/4 cup grated mozzarella cheese
Spritz a 2-quart pot with oil over medium heat and add 2 table-spoons tamari. Add onions and sauté until tamari is absorbed and onions are very soft. Add water, remaining tamari, sherry, and pepper. Heat to a slow boil and adjust seasonings to taste. Serve piping hot, topped with mozzarella cheese. Serves 4.

Lentil Soup

1 cup dry lentils
4 cups water
1 summer squash, finely chopped
1 zucchini, finely chopped
2 stalks celery, chopped
1–2 medium carrots, chopped
1 small onion, chopped
1 tsp salt (or to taste)
1 bay leaf
3 tbsp red wine vinegar (optional)
Bring water to a simmer in a large pot. Add lentils and cover, simmering gently for 1 hour. Stir in all other ingredients. Simmer uncovered until lentils are very soft. Add more water if needed, but soup should be thick. Serve hot. Serves 6.

Zucchini Soup

Spritzed oil
5 medium zucchini, chopped
1 large onion, chopped
2 large carrots, chopped
2 stalks celery, chopped
1–2 cups fresh peas, or 1 package (13-oz) frozen peas
1 tsp salt (or to taste)
1/2 tsp curry powder
1/2 tsp garlic powder
6–8 cups water

Spritz a large pot with oil over medium heat. Add onions, carrots, and celery and sauté until slightly tender. Add all other ingredients, cooking on moderate heat (but not boiling) until carrots are fully tender, about 20–30 minutes. Allow soup to cool slightly and then puree in a blender until not quite smooth. More pureeing will make a finer soup, but it should have some texture. Serve hot. Serves 8.

Split Pea Soup
1 cup dry green or yellow split peas
Tamari (to taste)
1 potato, peeled and diced
1 large onion, diced
4 garlic cloves, minced
2 stalks celery, diced
3 medium carrots, diced
1 large tomato, diced
3 tsp olive oil
2 tsp basil
2 tsp thyme
2 tsp no-salt vegetable broth
1 tbsp mustard
Freshly ground black pepper (to taste)
In a large pot of water, bring 8 cups of water to a rolling boil. Boil split peas and tamari, and add water as necessary as peas cook for 2-3 minutes. (Watch for sticking on the bottom of your soup pot.) Add potato to almost-cooked peas. In a separate pan, heat a small amount of oil over medium heat and sauté onion and garlic until onion is translucent. Add celery and carrot to pan and continue sautéing for 15 minutes. Add tomatoes, herbs, broth, and sautéed veggies to cooked peas, simmering 30 more minutes. Serves 6.

Gazpacho

2 tomatoes, finely diced
2 cucumbers, finely diced
1 green pepper, finely diced
1 (24-oz) can tomato juice
1 tsp Worcestershire sauce
1/2 tsp garlic powder
Juice of 1 lemon
Pinch ground black pepper
Pinch cayenne pepper
Combine all ingredients in a large bowl. Put half the mixture into a blender and puree until blended, then return to bowl. Stir to mix. Chill for several hours and serve cold. Serves 4.

Cold Melon Soup

1 ripe honeydew melon
1 ripe cantaloupe
3 large slices seeded watermelon
1 1/2 cups fresh pineapple chunks or 1 (8-oz) can unsweetened pineapple chunks
1 1/2 cups seltzer water
1 cup crushed ice
Fresh mint (for garnish)
Put all ingredients in a blender. Blend on high speed until smooth. Serve immediately, garnished with fresh mint. Serves 6-8.

Tropical Salsa

1 cup watermelon, cubed
1 cups fresh pineapple, diced
1/2 red onion, finely diced
1/2 green pepper, seeded and diced
1/4 cup fresh chives, chopped
1 tsp fresh ginger, finely diced
Juice from 1 orange

Juice from half a lime
1 tbsp honey
2–3 tbsp water to moisten
Combine all ingredients and set in refrigerator for 1 hour before serving. Makes 3 cups.

Salad Niçoise
1/2 lb green beans
1 lb baby spinach
1 (13-oz) can white tuna in water, drained
2 (5-inch) carrots, julienne sliced
1/2 lb greens
4 large mushroom caps, sliced
1 package alfalfa sprouts
2 hardboiled eggs, cut into quarters
Vinaigrette dressing
Cut ends off beans and steam until just tender. Remove from heat and chill for 2 or more hours. Arrange spinach in salad bowls or on plates. Put one-quarter of tuna in the center of each plate and arrange vegetables and egg quarters neatly around it. Serve with vinaigrette dressing. Serves 4.

Turkey or Chicken Curry Salad
1 cup unpeeled apples, cored and cubed
1 tsp lemon juice
8 oz cooked turkey or chicken breast, cubed
1/2 cup pineapple chunks
1/2 cup yogurt *
1/4 cup raisins
1/4 cup slivered almonds
1 tsp curry powder
Put apples in a large bowl with lemon juice to prevent them from turning brown. Add all other ingredients and mix well. Chill if desired. Serves 4-6.

* This is an example of how to use yogurt in a recipe that usually calls for mayonnaise. Remember, mayonnaise is about 80% fat while yogurt is only 30%, and there are 800 calories in a half cup of mayonnaise but only 62 calories in a half cup of yogurt.

Chicken Sesame and Spinach Pasta Salad
6 oz dry fusilli or rotini pasta
1/2 cup sesame seeds
1/2 cup light sesame or extra virgin olive oil
1/3 cup red wine vinegar
1/3 cup soy sauce
2 tbsp sugar
1/4 tsp pepper
3 cups cooked, shredded chicken
1/2 cup finely chopped parsley
1/2 cup thinly sliced green onion
8 cups (2 bunches) lightly packed fresh spinach, torn into pieces
Boil pasta, drain, and set aside. Heat 1/4 cup oil in a frying pan over medium heat and cook sesame seeds, stirring until golden. Cool. Stir in remaining oil, vinegar, soy sauce, sugar, and pepper. Pour over cooked pasta, adding chicken, and toss lightly. Cover and chill for at least 2 hours or overnight. To serve, add parsley, onions, and spinach. Toss gently.

Tabbouleh
2 cups water
1 cup bulghur
1 large ripe tomato, finely chopped
2 garlic cloves, crushed
1/4 cup fresh parsley, minced
1/4 cup fresh mint, minced
2 tbsp lemon juice
Lettuce leaves (for garnish)

Bring water to boil in a saucepan. Add bulghur, turn heat to low, cover, and simmer for 15 minutes or until done. Remove from heat and cool for 15 minutes. Transfer bulghur and all other ingredients into a large bowl, stirring with a fork to mix well. Chill for 4 hours or longer. Serve on a bed of lettuce. Makes 3 cups.

Hummus
2 cups cooked garbanzo beans or 2 (19-oz) cans garbanzo beans
2 garlic cloves, minced or 2 tsp garlic powder
Juice of 1 lemon
1 small red onion, diced
1 tomato, finely chopped
1 cucumber, finely chopped
Mash garbanzo beans in a medium bowl until smooth. Add garlic and lemon juice and mix well. Gently fold in onion, tomato, and cucumber. Makes 2 1/2 cups.

ENTRÉE RECIPES

Stuffed Chicken Roll-Up
1 6 oz chicken breast, trimmed of excess fat and pounded thin
4 stalks asparagus
2 oz part-skim mozzarella cheese, shredded

Sauce
6 oz chicken or turkey stock, divided
1 garlic clove, finely chopped
2 tsp freshly chopped rosemary
1 tsp cornstarch dissolved in 1 tsp water
Preheat oven to 350°F. Place cheese and asparagus at one end of breast and roll. Bake seam side down for approximately 15–18 minutes.

While chicken is baking, sauté garlic and rosemary in a saucepan over medium heat with 1 tablespoon of the stock. Add remaining stock, bring to a boil, and reduce heat to a simmer. Reduce for about 20 minutes and add cornstarch mixture, whisking until thickened. Simmer for 2 more minutes and spoon over Roll-up.

Stuffed Peppers
1/2 yellow onion, diced
1 garlic clove, diced
2 tbsp finely diced carrot
4 oz tofu
1/2 cup cooked lentils
1/2 cup cooked quinoa
Pinch fresh thyme and basil
1 tbsp grated Parmesan cheese
1 red bell pepper, seeded and halved
Preheat oven to 350°F. Sauté onion, garlic, carrot, and tofu in a medium non-stick pan over medium heat. Add fresh herbs and continue to cook for another minute. Remove pan from heat and stir in all remaining ingredients, except bell pepper. Stuff pepper halves with mixture and bake for 25 minutes. Serves 2.

New Life Salmon Cakes

Salmon Cakes
1 1/2 lb cooked salmon, flaked
5 tbsp light mayonnaise
2 celery stalks, minced
2 tbsp fresh parsley, chopped
1 egg yolk
Juice of half a lemon
1 1/2 tbsp Old Bay Seasoning
1/2 tsp salt
Ground black pepper (to taste)

2 cups fresh breadcrumbs
3 tbsp olive oil

Horseradish Sauce
1 1/2 cups low fat yogurt
2 tbsp horseradish, drained
Juice of half a lemon
1 tbsp hot sauce
2 tbsp fresh dill, coarsely chopped
Salt (to taste)
Mix all ingredients for horseradish sauce together in a medium bowl. Refrigerate sauce while preparing salmon cakes. Mix ingredients for salmon cakes together in a large bowl, except breadcrumbs and oil. Stir 1 cup fresh breadcrumbs into the mixture, and then spread remaining cup of breadcrumbs on a large plate. Shape salmon mixture into 8 cakes, pressing firmly to ensure the cakes hold their shape. Coat each salmon cake with breadcrumbs, pressing lightly for an even coat. Heat oil in a large skillet over medium heat. Place salmon cakes into skillet and cook about 2 minutes on each side until brown. Serves 4.

Salmon en Papilote
2 (4–6 oz) salmon filets
Your choice of: onion, celery, red and green peppers, snow peas, carrot, asparagus, scallion, kale, spinach
2 tsp white wine
Garlic powder (to taste)
Paprika (to taste)
Ground black pepper (to taste)
2 lemon wedges
2 fresh sprigs of dill or tarragon
Preheat oven to 350°F. Cut 2 pieces of parchment paper measuring 10 × 12 inches. Make a neat pile with your vegetables of choice in the center of each parchment sheet. Lay salmon filets

over the vegetables and drizzle with white wine, then sprinkle with seasonings. Be gentle. Less is more. Lay lemon slice on top, then the herb sprig. Fold the parchement over to make a pocket and crinkle the edges up to create a half circle. Bake for 20–25 minutes. Tear open and enjoy! Serves 2.

Baked Stuffed Shrimp
12 large shrimp, peeled and deveined
1 tbsp onion, finely diced
1 tbsp celery, finely diced
Zest and juice of one lemon
Zest and juice of one lime
3 tbsp wheat germ or breadcrumbs
1 tbsp fresh parsley, chopped
2 (6.5-oz) cans baby clams or crabmeat, chopped
1 tbsp coconut flakes
1 tbsp Parmesan cheese
1 egg
1 garlic clove, crushed
1 tsp Old Bay Seasoning
Ground black pepper to taste
Preheat oven to 350°F. To butterfly shrimp, slice the underneath of the body lengthwise and fold open. Mix all remaining ingredients together in a large mixing bowl to prepare stuffing. Roll a small ball of stuffing in your palm. Wrap one shrimp around the stuffing and place on a baking sheet with the tails on top. Bake for 25–30 minutes. Serves 4.

Shrimp Fantasia
1 tsp dark toasted sesame oil
2 scallions, chopped
4 garlic cloves, minced
2 tsp fresh ginger, peeled and chopped

1 1/2 tsp mild curry paste (a good one is Patak's mild) or 1/2 tsp each (cumin, chili powder, and coriander)
1 lb shrimp (about 20), thawed and deveined
4 medium plum tomatoes, diced small
1/4 cup freshly chopped basil
Freshly ground black pepper
Tamari (to taste)
Heat sesame oil in large skillet over medium heat and sauté scallions, garlic, ginger, and curry paste for 2 minutes. Add shrimp and cook for 2 minutes. Add tomatoes, basil, pepper and tamari. Cook on medium heat until shrimp are done and tomatoes are heated through. Serves 4–5.

Salmon with Creamy Tomato Sauce
4 (4–6 oz) salmon filets
1/4 cup soy-ginger marinade
1/4 cup white wine
Scallions, chopped
Fresh dill, chopped
Fresh thyme, chopped
Fresh tarragon, chopped

Creamy Tomato Sauce
Spritzed oil
1/4 medium onion, finely diced
3 garlic cloves, minced
1/2 tsp dill
1/4 tsp thyme (use 2x fresh if available)
Freshly ground black pepper (to taste)
2 tsp low fat cream cheese or Neufchatel
3 medium plum tomatoes, medium diced
Tamari (to taste)
1 tsp cornstarch in 1 tbsp water (if necessary)

Preheat oven to 350°F. If possible, marinate salmon 15 minutes before cooking. Place salmon on baking sheet, drizzle with liquids, and dress with fresh herbs. Bake for 15–20 minutes. Near the end of the cooking time, check the salmon often for doneness. This dish can be pan cooked as well.

While salmon is baking, spritz a saucepan with oil over medium heat and sauté onion and garlic. Add herbs, pepper, cream cheese, and tomatoes. Sweat over medium heat until heated through but not yet mushy. Adjust thickness with cornstarch mixture, if necessary. Add tamari to taste. Serve immediately over poached salmon. Serves 4.

Seafood Kabobs

1 lb fresh swordfish, cut into 1 1/2-inch cubes
1/2 lb scallops or shrimp
2 green peppers, cut into large chunks
6 large mushrooms
6 cherry tomatoes
1 small eggplant, cut into large chunks
2 Vidalia onions, cut into large chunks
Spritzed oil
6 lemon wedges (optional)

Arrange seafood and vegetables in any combination on 6 wooden kabob skewers. Spritz each kabob with a little oil and grill slowly for about 15 minutes, turning every 3–4 minutes. Baking the kabobs on a pan in the oven at 325°F for 25—30 minutes is also an option. Serve with fresh lemon wedges. Makes 6 kabobs.

Savory Tuna

4 (6-oz) tuna steaks, trimmed of skin, rinsed, and dried
1/2 tsp lime zest
1 garlic clove, crushed
2 tsp olive oil
1 tsp ground cumin

1 tsp ground coriander
Ground black pepper (to taste)
1 tsp lime juice
Fresh cilantro (for garnish)
In a small bowl, combine lime zest, garlic, olive oil, cumin, coriander and pepper into a paste. Spread paste thinly on both sides of tuna steaks. Heat a nonstick griddle pan over medium-high heat and press steaks into skillet to seal them. Lower heat and cook for 5 minutes. Turn over, cook an additional 4–5 minutes until cooked through. Drain on paper towels and transfer to a warmed serving plate. Sprinkle lime juice and chopped cilantro on top. Serves 4.

Grilled Swordfish
2 cups apple-raspberry juice or your favorite mixed-fruit juice
Juice of 3 oranges
Juice of 2 lemons
Juice of 1 lime
1 tbsp minced parsley
1 1/2 tsp fresh basil
1 tsp marjoram
1 1/2 lb swordfish, cut into 6-oz portions
4 lemon wedges (for garnish)
Mix juice and spices in a large bowl. Add swordfish and marinate for 24 hours. Grill over open flame for 15 minutes, turning every 3–4 minutes. Serve with a lemon wedge. Serves 4.

Oat-Crusted Chicken
1/2 cup rolled oats
1 tbsp fresh, chopped rosemary
Paprika (to taste)
Ground black pepper (to taste)
1 garlic clove, crushed
2 whole eggs

4 boneless, skinless chicken breasts

Sauce
2/3 cup nonfat plain yogurt
2 tsp wholegrain mustard
2 tsp honey
Preheat oven to 350°F. Combine oats, rosemary, paprika, pepper, and garlic in a shallow bowl. Beat eggs and brush each chicken breast with egg mixture, then coat with oat mixture. Place the chicken pieces on a baking sheet and bake for 30–35 minutes. While chicken is baking, combine yogurt, mustard, and honey to make sauce. Spoon sauce over chicken and season with pepper before serving. Serves 4.

Flank Steak Kabob
2 cups soy sauce
1 tbsp fresh, minced ginger
1 tbsp fresh, minced garlic
Juice of 2 oranges
1 tbsp cornstarch mixed with 1 tbsp water
6-oz flank steak, pounded thin
In a small saucepan over medium heat, bring soy sauce, ginger, garlic, and juice to a simmer. Whisk in cornstarch mixture. Bring to a boil and simmer until sauce thickens.

Marinate flank steak for 1–2 hours and skewer the long way. Grill to desired doneness.

Teriyaki Chicken
4 boneless, skinless chicken breasts
2 cups tamari
1 cup Worcestershire
Juice from 1 8 oz. can of pineapple
2 garlic cloves, crushed
Zest and juice of 2 oranges

Zest and juice of 1 lemon
3 cups water
Ground black pepper (to taste)
Combine all ingredients in a large bowl. Marinate chicken breasts in sauce for 2 hours or more. Grill 7–8 minutes on each side or until cooked through. Serves 4

Chicken Dijon
Spritzed oil
4 boneless, skinless chicken breasts
1/8 cup white wine
1 1/2 tsp cornstarch mixed with 1 1/2 tbsp water (optional)

Dijon Sauce
1 tbsp olive oil
1 medium onion, diced
2 garlic cloves, minced
1/4 tsp basil
1/4 tsp thyme
Ground black pepper (to taste)
3/4 cup 1% milk
1 tbsp low-fat cream cheese or Neufchâtel
Wholegrain mustard (to taste)
To make the Dijon sauce, heat oil in a large saucepan over medium heat and sauté onion until clear. Add garlic and spices and sauté for a few more minutes. Stir in milk and pour sauce mixture into a blender with cream cheese. Puree into a thin (not watery) sauce. Return to saucepan and simmer on low heat. Add mustard to taste. Adjust with milk if too thick. To make the chicken, spritz a skillet with oil over medium-high heat. Add chicken breasts and adjust heat to achieve a quick browning of both sides. Add white wine to deglaze skillet. Simmer chicken in Dijon sauce until the breasts are cooked through, about 10 minutes. If sauce is too thin, thicken with

half the cornstarch mixture, simmering for one minute and adding slowly until desired consistency is reached. Serves 4.

Chicken or Tofu Satay

4 boneless, skinless chicken breasts or 1 package extra-firm tofu, sliced into steaks

Marinade

1/4 cup vegetable stock
1/4 cup light coconut milk
1 1/2 tbsp mild curry paste
1 tsp fresh ginger
1 tsp turmeric

Satay Sauce

1/2 cup hot water
1/2 cup peanut butter
1/4 cup coconut milk
2 tbsp honey
2 tbsp tamari
1 tbsp tamarind
1 tbsp lime zest
4 lime slices (for garnish)

Combine marinade ingredients in a large bowl and marinate chicken or tofu for 2 hours. Combine satay sauce ingredients in a separate bowl and brush sauce over chicken or tofu before grilling. Grill chicken 7–8 minutes on each side or until cooked through. Grill tofu steaks 3–4 minutes each side. Serve with a slice of lime. Serves 4.

Spanakopita

16 sheets of filo dough, completely defrosted

Filling
1/2 cup olive oil, divided
2 cups minced onion
1 tsp fresh basil
1 tsp fresh oregano
2 1/2 tbsp stemmed and finely chopped fresh spinach
4 garlic cloves. minced
2 tbsp flour
2 1/2 cups crumbled feta cheese
1 cup cottage cheese
Ground black pepper (to taste)

Preheat oven to 375°F. Heat 1 tablespoon oil in a large sauté pan over medium heat. Add onions, garlic, and herbs and sauté for 5 minutes, or until the onions are soft. Add the spinach, stirring frequently so it doesn't stick. Cook until the spinach wilts. Sprinkle in flour, stir, and cook over medium heat 2–3 minutes. Remove from heat and mix in the cheeses. Taste and adjust flavor accordingly. Oil a 9 × 13-inch baking pan and unwrap filo dough. Place a sheet of filo on the oiled pan. Brush lightly with remaining oil, and then add another sheet. Continue this process until you have used 8 sheets of dough. Add the filling to the pan and spread evenly. Layer the rest of dough on top of the filling in the same manner as the first 8 sheets. Oil the top layer and bake for about 45 minutes or until crispy. Cut into squares, and serve hot or warm. Makes 6 entrée servings or 24 appetizer servings.

Spaghetti Squash Pizza Crust
3 cups cooked spaghetti squash
2 eggs, beaten
2 1/2 cups shredded part-skim mozzarella cheese, divided
2–3 tbsp pizza sauce
1 tbsp freshly chopped oregano
3 tbsp freshly chopped basil

Assorted vegetables or other toppings

Preheat oven to 400°F. Squeeze the excess moisture out of the cooked spaghetti squash with paper towels. Mix the squash, eggs, and 1 1/2 cups mozzarella together. Press the mixture into the bottom of a pie pan. Bake for about 10 minutes. Remove the pan from the oven and spread the tomato sauce, vegetables or other pizza toppings, and the remaining cheese over the crust. Sprinkle with oregano and basil and drizzle the olive oil over the top. Bake for 25 minutes or until cheese is lightly browned.

Vegetarian Lasagna

1 (16-oz) box whole wheat pasta

4 cups tomato sauce

2 cups lightly wilted spinach or frozen spinach, thawed and drained

1/2 lb firm tofu

1 cup part-skim ricotta cheese

1 tbsp minced garlic

1/2 tbsp dried oregano

1/2 tbsp dried basil

Ground black pepper (to taste)

1/2 cup Parmesan cheese

1 cup part-skim mozzarella cheese

Preheat oven to 350°F. Cook noodles al dente (firm but soft) and set aside to cool. Mix tofu, ricotta cheese, garlic, oregano, basil, and pepper in a medium bowl. In a baking dish, place a small amount of tomato sauce, followed by one layer of noodles. Spread one-third of the cheese mixture over the noodles and top with one-third of the wilted spinach. Repeat the layers 2 more times and cover the final layer of noodles with remaining sauce. Sprinkle mozzarella and Parmesan over the top. Bake for 45–55 minutes until cheese is bubbly and lightly browned. Serves 8.

Baked Sweet Potatoes

2 lb sweet potatoes, peeled and cubed

1 cup unsweetened fruit juice

1/4 cup Vermont maple syrup

1 tsp fresh, grated ginger

1/2 tsp ground cinnamon

1/4 tsp ground cardamom

1/4 tsp tamari

Preheat oven to 350°F. Place sweet potatoes in 8 cups boiling water and simmer for 5 minutes. In a large baking dish, stir together juice, syrup, ginger, cinnamon, cardamom and tamari. Drain potatoes and add to baking dish, coating with the juice mixture. Bake uncovered for 1 hour, stirring every 15 minutes until potatoes are tender and juice has thickened. Serves 4.

DESSERT RECIPES

Berry Berry Crisp

6 oz blueberries

6 oz blackberries

6 oz raspberries

2 lemons, halved

1/2 cup dry quick oats

1 tbsp wheat germ

4 tbsp honey or maple syrup

Pinch cinnamon

Pinch nutmeg

Preheat oven to 350°F. Divide berry varieties between 4 small oven-safe bowls, mixing gently. Squeeze the juice from half a lemon over each bowl. Combine oats, wheat germ, syrup, and spice in a separate bowl and sprinkle a small amount on top of each berry mixture. Place the bowls in a 2-inch deep baking dish and fill about a half inch with water to make a "water bath." Place pan in the oven and bake for 45 minutes.

Chocolate Chippers
1 1/4 cup whole wheat pastry flour
2/3 cup turbinado
1 tsp baking soda
1/4 cup prune puree
2 tbsp honey
1 tsp vanilla
1/3 cup chocolate chips
1/3 cup walnuts
Fruit juice (as needed)
Preheat oven to 350°F. Mix dry ingredients together in a large bowl and then add wet ingredients. If dough is dry, add small amounts of fruit juice to moisten. Place small balls on a cookie sheet, spaced 2 inches apart, and bake for 12–15 minutes. Makes 6 cookies.

New Life Sundaes
4 perfectly ripe bananas, sliced
Chocolate sauce
Nuts and berries (optional)
Freeze sliced bananas in a plastic bag. Remove from freezer, thaw 10 minutes, and then place in blender. Puree until smooth. Consistency will be like ice cream. Use a bit of vanilla yogurt or part of an unfrozen ripe banana in blender to thicken, if needed. Top with chocolate sauce, nuts, and berries. Serves 4.

Chocolate Sauce
2/3 cup 1% milk or water
1/3 cup maple syrup
2 1/2 tbsp cocoa powder

2 tsp cornstarch

2 tbsp water

1/2 tsp vanilla, mocha, or some other flavored extract

In a small saucepan combine first 3 ingredients and bring to a low boil. Blend together cornstarch and water in a small bowl and drizzle gradually into saucepan, simmering a few seconds and stirring constantly. Adjust thickness if necessary. Add vanilla or other flavored extract.

Berry Parfait with Orange-Custard Sauce

2 strips orange peel

1 1/2 cups skim milk

2 eggs, lightly beaten

1/4 cup clover or orange blossom honey

1/2 tsp vanilla

2 cups sliced strawberries

1 tbsp sugar

1 tbsp Cointreau or Grand Marnier (optional)

1/2 tsp grated orange zest

Fresh berries (optional)

With vegetable peeler, cut 2 wide strips of orange peel (orange part only) and add to milk. Heat milk with peels in small saucepan (or in microwave about 3 minutes) until hot but not boiling. Meanwhile, in top part of a double boiler, whisk together eggs and honey. Gradually add heated milk to egg mixture, stirring constantly. Set mixture over simmering water and cook on low heat, stirring constantly until mixture coats a metal spoon (about 10–15 minutes). Remove from heat. Remove orange peel and add vanilla. Cool and layer with fresh berries. Chill. 4 servings.

Super Moist Apple Cake

2 cups whole wheat pastry flour

1/2 cup turbinado

1 tsp baking soda

Cinnamon or nutmeg (optional)
3/4 cup apple juice
1 tsp vanilla extract
2 cups finely chopped apples
1/2 cup raisins or walnuts
Spritzed oil
Combine dry ingredients in a large bowl. Add juice and vanilla, stirring until dry mixture is just moistened. Fold in apples and raisins or walnuts. Spritz an 8 × 4-inch loaf pan with oil. Spread mixture evenly in pan and bake at 325°F for 50 minutes. Remove bread from oven and let stand for 10 minutes in pan. Invert onto a wire rack or serving board and slice once completely cool.

Lemon Ricotta
1 cup part-skim ricotta cheese
1/2 tsp grated lemon peel
1/2 tsp vanilla extract
2 tbsp clover or orange blossom honey
Fresh berries or kiwi
Mix the ricotta cheese, lemon peel, vanilla extract, and honey. Serve chilled with fresh berries or kiwi. Serves 2–4.

Chocolate Pie
1/3 cup maple syrup
2/3 cup milk or water
4 tbsp cocoa powder
2 tbsp cornstarch
1/8 cup cold water
3 eggs
1 tsp vanilla
2 cups of any of the following:
Nonfat or regular cottage cheese
Nonfat or regular ricotta cheese

Preheat the oven to 325°F. Mix first 3 ingredients in a 1-quart saucepan and bring to a simmer. Make a slurry with cornstarch and cold water. Add slurry to pan, simmering and stirring mixture for 1 minute until thickened. Use whisk if necessary. Combine thickened sauce with last 3 ingredients in blender until silky smooth. Pour mixture into 8-inch pie pan and bake for approximately 1 hour and 15 minutes, checking for doneness after about 1 hour. Chill for at least 1 hour and 30 minutes before serving. Serves 6.

Bibliography

Epigraph
"Destination Spa Group: Summer Words of Wellness." Posted May 19, 2013. *Spafinder Wellness Blog.* https://www.spafinder.com/blog/spa-travel/destination-spa-group-summer-words-wellness/

Your Journey to Wellness
Carroll, Aaron E. "To Lose Weight, Eating Less Is Far More Important Than Exercising More." Posted June 15, 2015. *New York Times.* https://www.nytimes.com/2015/06/16/upshot/to-lose-weight-eating-less-is-far-more-important-than-exercising-more.html?_r=0.

Ferdman, Roberto A. "Why Diets Don't Actually Work, According to a Researcher Who Has Studied Them for Decades." Posted May 4, 2015. *Washington Post.* https://www.washingtonpost.com/news/wonk/wp/2015/05/04/why-diets-dont-actually-work-according-to-a-researcher-who-has-studied-them-for-decades/?utm_term=.a806fb902b25.

Simple Steps for Every Day
"Natural Peanut Butter vs. Regular Peanut Butter." Posted July 8, 2013. RealHealth. https://www.realhealthmag.com/article/peanutbutter-health-transfats-24167-3676.

Yoquinto, Luke. "The Truth about Food Additive BHA." Posted June 1, 2012. LiveScience. https://www.livescience.com/36424-food-additive-bha-butylated-hydroxyanisole.html.

"EWG's Dirty Dozen Guide to Food Additives." Posted November 12, 2014. *Environmental Working Group*. http://www. ewg.org/research/ewg-s-dirty-dozen-guide-food-additives/ generally-recognized-as-safe-but-is-it.

Nirenberg, Carl. "New Health Warning Explained: How Processed Meat Is Linked to Cancer." Posted October 30, 2015. *LiveScience*. https://www.livescience.com/52651-red-meat-cancer-warning-explained.html.

Billings-Smith, Lana. "What Is Potassium Sorbate." Updated April 23. 2015. *Livestrong*. http://www.livestrong.com/ article/31559-potassium-sorbate/.

Orciari, Megan. "Compulsive Eating and Substance Dependence Share Similar Brain Patterns." Posted April 4, 2011. *YaleNews*. https://news.yale.edu/2011/04/04/compulsive-eating-and-substance-dependence-share-similar-brain-patterns.

Spend Time in Nature Exercising
LeWine, Howard, MD. "Benefits of Vitamin D Supplements Still Debated." Posted April 4, 2014. *Harvard Health Publications*. http://www.health.harvard.edu/blog/benefits-vitamin-d-supp lements-still-debated-201404047106.

Reynolds, Gretchen. "The Benefits of Exercising Outdoors." Posted February 21, 2013. *New York Times*. https://well.blogs.nytimes. com/2013/02/21/the-benefits-of-exercising-outdoors/?_r=0.

Thompson, Coon J., K. Boddy, K. Stein, R. Whear, J. Barton, and M. H. Depledge. "Does Participating in Physical Activity in Outdoor Natural Environments Have a a Greater Effect on Physical and Mental Wellbeing than Physical Activity Indoors? A Systematic Review." Posted March 1, 2011. *Environmental Science & Technology.* https://www.ncbi.nlm.nih.gov/pubmed/21291246.

Sutton, Amy. "Calories Burned When Walking on Different Surfaces." Chron. http://livehealthy.chron.com/calories-burned-walking-different-surfaces-4734.html

"Memory Improved 20% by Nature Walk." Psyblog. http://www.spring.org.uk/2009/01/memory-improved-20-by-nature-walk.php.

Hartig, Terry., Marlis Mang, and Gary W. Evans. "Restorative Effects of Natural Environment Experiences." *Environment and Behavior.* http://journals.sagepub.com/doi/abs/10.1177/00139 16591231001.

The Truth about Your Metabolism
Sifferlin, Alexandra. "Stressful Days Can Slow Your Metabolism, Study Says." Posted July 14, 2014. *Time Health.* http://time.com/2981436/women-stress-eating-11-pounds/.

Jensen, Pernille. "The Chemicals That Can Affect Your Metabolism." Updated October 8, 2016. *HuffPost Blog.* http://www.huffingtonpost.com/pernille-jensen/the-chemicals-that-affect_b_8218034.html.

Adams, Jill U. "Are Parabens and Phthalates Harmful in Makeup and Lotion?" Posted September 1, 2014. *Washington Post.* https://www.washingtonpost.com/national/health-science/are-parabens-and-phthalates-harmful-in-makeup-and-lotions/2014/08/29/

aa7f9d34-2c6f-11e4-994d-202962a9150c_story. html?utm_term=.3aec1213f8fa.

Benefits of Massage and Bodywork
"9 Scientifically Proven Health Benefits of Massage." *Morgan Massage Blog.* http://morganmassage.com/2012/12/09/9-health-benefits-of-massage/.

Hsu, Matt. "What Does Rolfing Have to Do with Emotions?" Posted March 30, 2008. Rolfing. http://align.org/2008/03/30/what-does-rolfing-have-to-do-with-emotions/.

Database of Christian massage therapists: http://christianmassage.org/.

Benefits of Quiet Time
Achor, Shawn. "Why You Need that 5 Minutes of Quiet." Posted July 22, 2014. Good Housekeeping. http://www.goodhousekeeping.com/health/wellness/advice/a25603/health-benefits-quiet.

Benefits of Fasting
Bair, Stephanie. "Intermittent Fasting: Try This at Home for Brain Health." Posted January 9, 2015. *Stanford Law School Law and Biosciences Blog.* https://law.stanford.edu/2015/01/09/lawandbiosciences-2015-01-09-intermittent-fasting-try-this-at-home-for-brain-health/.

Benefits of Essential Oils
"13 Surprising Benefits of Lavender Essential Oil." Organic Facts. https://www.organicfacts.net/health-benefits/essential-oils/health-benefits-of-lavender-essential-oil.html.

The Benefits of a "Natural Wrapper Diet"

"21 Amazing Things that Happen to Your Body When You Eat Bananas." Eat This, Not That! http://www.eatthis.com/benefits-of-bananas.

Dennis, Adonia. "Health News: How Grapes Can Help Cut Down the Risk of Obesity." Posted May 23, 2016. HuffPost Blog. http://www.huffingtonpost.com/adonia-dennis/how-grapes-can-help-you-c_b_10062028.html.

Cooper, Belle Beth. "Novelty and the Brain: Why New Things Make Us Feel So Good." Posted May 21, 2013. Lifehacker. https://lifehacker.com/novelty-and-the-brain-why-new-things-make-us-feel-so-g-508983802

Surround Yourself with Good People
Bradberry, Travis. "How Successful People Handle Toxic People." Posted October 21, 2014. Forbes. https://www.forbes.com/sites/travisbradberry/2014/10/21/how-successful-people-handle-toxic-people/#609fba282a92.

Downing, Carla. "Christian Relationship Devotional: Necessary Endings." Change My Relationship. http://www.changemyrelationship.com/christian-relationship-devotional-necessary-endings/.

Target Your Habits for Lasting Wellness
Brynie, Faith, PhD. "Food and the Brain's Reward System." Posted August 15, 2013. Psychology Today. https://www.psychologytoday.com/blog/brain-sense/201308/food-and-the-brains-reward-system.

About the Author

Kathleen LeSage is a Certified Health Coach, the owner of the trademark "The Natural Wrapper Diet" and co-owns with her husband one of America's top destination spa and wellness retreats.

Kathleen has appeared on A&E's *It's a Living* and *Good Morning America*. She held a career in public relations and marketing, working with such companies as Marriott International and Woodward & Lothrop in Washington, DC.

For the past fifteen years she has run New Life Hiking Spa with her husband. Under Kathleen's marketing management, New Life has won the #1 Destination Spa of 2016 by Travel + Leisure magazine and appeared on the Today Show. New Life has become one of the best-known wellness retreats in North America and has been featured in Health magazine, AARP The Magazine, Shape magazine, SELF magazine, Rand McNally and USA Today. Kathleen currently resides with her husband and two children in Vermont and Florida, where they all do their part in running the family business. They enjoy traveling, homeschooling, and outdoor activities in which they can just appreciate God's amazing creation.